The Angry Gut

Coping with Colitis and Crohn's Disease

OTHER BOOKS BY W. GRANT THOMPSON

Gut Reactions (Plenum Press, New York, New York: 1989)
The Irritable Gut (University Park Press, Baltimore, Maryland: 1979)

The Angry Gut
Coping with Colitis and Crohn's Disease

W. Grant Thompson, M.D.

Plenum Press • New York and London

Library of Congress Cataloging-in-Publication Data

Thompson, W. Grant.
    The angry gut : coping with colitis and Crohn's disease / W. Grant
  Thompson.
        p.   cm.
    Includes bibliographical references and index.
    ISBN 0-306-44470-4
    1. Inflammatory bowel diseases.   I. Title.
    [DNLM: 1. Colitis, Ulcerative.   2. Crohn Disease.   3. Inflammatory
  Bowel Diseases.   WI 522 T478a]
  RC862.I53T49   1993
  616.3'44--dc20
  DNLM/DLC
  for Library of Congress   92-48259
                                                                        CIP

The treatments outlined in this volume are intended to serve only as examples.
You should consult your personal physician before beginning any medical
treatment regimen.

Chapters 1 and 2 are adapted from the author's *Gut Reactions,*
published by Plenum Press in 1989.

ISBN 0-306-44470-4

Printed in the United States of America

To
my patients,
whose fortitude in adversity
is a daily inspiration

Preface

An inflamed gut is an angry gut. Inflammation is a means by which the body defends itself against an infection or other noxious agent. In inflammatory bowel disease (IBD), the affected gut becomes hot, angry red, swollen, and painful. Unlike the acute, short-lived inflammation seen with infections such as salmonella, that of IBD is chronic and of unknown cause. Thus, the angry gut vents its wrath against an unknown assailant through abdominal pain, diarrhea, and the impedimenta of chronic illness. *Inflammatory bowel disease* is a generic term used to embrace two chronic manifestations of the angry gut—ulcerative colitis and Crohn's disease.

Inflammatory bowel disease characteristically afflicts the young, and its consequences may be a lifetime burden. It is not a killer, but it may temporarily disable; at best, it is a major inconvenience. Perhaps because it is seldom fatal, or because its symptoms are not suitable topics for polite conversation, IBD is not so well known as many less common diseases. Yet, because of the disability and suffering it causes, IBD deserves much more public attention. The inflammatory bowel diseases, Crohn's disease and ulcerative colitis, are complicated processes of unknown cause, unpredictable course, and trial-and-error treatment. To those who must deal with them— as patients, as spouses, as parents, or as professionals—these diseases seem formidable, even foreboding. Clearly explaining the angry gut to the newly afflicted is difficult, and fraught with caveats, because it may manifest in such a variety of ways. Yet much is known about IBD, and knowledge can comfort. Sufferers can do much to help themselves once they understand their disease.

This book is intended for patients with IBD, their families, and the nurses, primary care physicians, and other health professionals who are called on to help. It is not intended as a textbook for gastroenterologists or surgeons; other volumes fulfill that role. I have tried to simplify the medical terminology, and use plain English in place of medical jargon when suitable words exist. Some concepts in IBD are complicated, however. Although my purpose is to explain the angry gut to the literate lay reader, the subject does not permit oversimplification for easy comprehension. Opinions expressed here are derived from my experience as a gastroenterologist and clinical teacher.

Some basic information is necessary to understand IBD. In Part One, the relevant anatomy and physiology of the gut are described for those with no medical training. These two chapters are adapted for *The Angry Gut* from my previous book, *Gut Reactions*. Chapter Three introduces the vocabulary of IBD. Although they are considered twentieth-century diseases, examination of the older literature indicates that ulcerative colitis and Crohn's disease existed in the nineteenth century and probably before. The particularly great prevalence and incidence of IBD in people originating in Western Europe is tantalizing information, but despite much research, the cause remains a mystery. These matters are also discussed in Part One.

Parts Two and Three describe ulcerative colitis and Crohn's disease, respectively. Although they have many similarities, they are also very different from each other, and the differences are highlighted in these two parts. The distinct pathologies explain the different manifestations of the two diseases. Despite some similarities in treatment, the therapy particular to each disease is discussed in Chapters Nine and Thirteen, respectively. The complications, described in these parts, are also distinct.

A number of other topics (germane to IBD) that merit discussion are covered in Part Four. *Variant* colitis may be related to, or confused with, IBD. Both ulcerative colitis and Crohn's disease have associated extraintestinal manifestations or associated diseases that, on occasion, are more troubling than the intestinal disease itself. Also, the relationship of ulcerative colitis to colon cancer becomes ominous over time and necessitates preventive intervention. The risks and options are discussed in Chapter Seventeen. Most important, these diseases may adversely affect one's quality of life. The psychosocial, sexual, and reproductive implications of IBD are difficult to quantify, but as described at the end of Part Four, they now receive the attention they deserve. Whereas physicians necessarily focus on the physical manifestations of an angry gut, patients' concerns center on daily functioning.

Part Five consists of more detailed discussions of the therapeutics, nutrition, and surgery employed in IBD. Each has a role in the management plan, and one must understand their good and bad effects. The last chapter describes some tests that the patient with IBD might expect to undergo; the purpose is to demystify them. Comprehension of the indications for and technique of a test may reduce fear and anxiety in those who must submit to it.

Finally, an angry gut is best managed when the patient is in partnership with a caring physician who is knowledgeable and experienced in treating ulcerative colitis and Crohn's disease. No amount of reading will produce an expert, and experience with the many twists and turns of these unpredictable diseases is essential to optimal care. So also is an informed patient. Treatment works best when the patient understands the disease and can actively participate in therapy under the physician's guidance. There is no quick fix—IBD, although manageable, just keeps coming back. This book aims to equip patients, their families, and health care workers to enter into an intelligent partnership with the physician. As with all human endeavors, communication is essential, and understanding, a prerequisite.

W. Grant Thompson

Mt. Tremblant, Quebec, Canada

Acknowledgments

Several colleagues helped me with various parts of the manuscript. They include Dr. D. G. Patel, Dr. H. Tao, Dr. M. Guindi, and Dr. J. R. Barr of the University of Ottawa, Dr. Paul Belliveau of McGill University, and Dr. D. A. Drossman of the University of North Carolina. Responsibility for any shortcomings, however, is solely mine.

Mr. James Harbinson prepared the illustrations, and Dr. Tao helped me select the radiographs. Mrs. Helen Kierczak assisted with final preparation of the manuscript.

This endeavor would not have been possible without the love and support of my wife Susan, who had to compete with Word-Perfect to get the chores done. The inspiration for the book is my patients. The manner in which they cope with the adversity of IBD, yet carry on useful work and productive family lives, is a model any artist might envy.

Contents

xiii

PART ONE

Understanding Inflammatory Bowel Disease

CHAPTER ONE

The Gut: A Brief Anatomy

Anatomy is to physiology as geography is to history; it is the theatre of
events.

Jean Fernel (1497–1558)

Gut is an Anglo-Saxon word that covers the subject from mouth to
anus. *Intestine*, like many Franco-English words, may appeal to the
sensitive, but it excludes the stomach and the esophagus. *Bowel* and
intestine refer only to the lower part. The *digestive*, *alimentary*, or
gastrointestinal tract may get around some of these difficulties but
excludes the pancreas and liver. These terms are seldom used
outside medical meetings. Perhaps the word gut is less objection-
able now, because it is the title of a distinguished British medical
journal. This chapter briefly outlines the anatomy of the gut, all
segments of which may be affected by inflammatory bowel disease
(IBD). No attempt is made to describe the gut in the detail required
by physicians and surgeons.

HISTOLOGY

Like all living tissue, the gut is made up of cells. The study of
cellular tissue is called *histology* and must be carried out through a
microscope. Histology of the gut is very complex (Figures 1-1 and

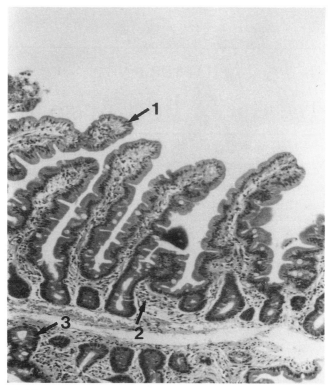

Figure 1-1. Photomicrograph of luminal side or mucosa of small-intestine wall. (1) Epithelium lining tall villi which project into the gut lumen. (2) Mucosa. Note the many cell nuclei. These are principally inflammatory or immune-competent cells, essential defenses against foreign invaders. (3) Crypts where epithelial cell reproduction occurs.

1-2). The single layer of cells lining the gut is called the epithelium. Under this epithelial cell layer is the mucosa, which contains a variety of cells important in the local immune and chemical reactions to gut injury. These cells include polymorphonuclear leukocytes (multinucleated white blood cells) and mononuclear cells such as lymphocytes, plasma cells, and macrophages, all of which participate in the immune response should any foreign substance

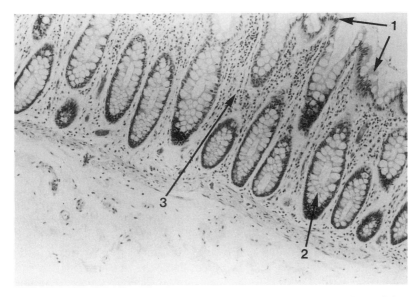

Figure 1-2. Photomicrograph of luminal side or mucosa of colon wall. (1) Colon epithelium lining the gut lumen. (2) Crypts. (3) Mucosa rich in inflammatory and immune-competent cells.

invade their territory. Notable among the remaining cells are those of nerve plexuses, blood vessels, and chemical-producing cells, such as mast cells. A thin muscle layer (muscularis mucosae) separates the mucosa from its supporting submucosa. Under the submucosa are the muscle and serosal layers of the gut. In the mucosa and submucosa, rich with immune cells, the gut's ongoing battle with its internal foreign environment takes place. As we shall see, it is here that IBD begins.

STRUCTURE OF THE GUT

At autopsy the human gut is 9 meters (30 feet) from mouth to anus. In the living person, the gut muscle tone contracts it to about one half of that length. Although the mouth and throat are part of the gut, our story begins at the esophagus (gullet), and continues through the stomach, small intestine, colon, rectum, and anus. The esophagus, stomach, small bowel, and colon are arranged within the chest and abdominal cavity as shown in Figure 1-3. The gut is a hollow, very flexible tube, the wall of which has three layers: an outer coating called the *serosa*, a muscular layer called the *muscularis*, and an inner lining called the *mucosa* (Figure 1-4).

The gut is a dynamic organ almost always on the move, and the driving force is the gut muscle. There are two muscle coats. The outer, thinner layer consists of muscle cells or fibers arranged in a longitudinal manner. In the colon, this layer becomes three longitudinal bands called *taenia coli*. The longitudinal layer shortens and lengthens as the gut moves its contents along. The inner, circular layer becomes thickened or specialized at various points to form one-way valves or *sphincters*. Circular and longitudinal muscle contractions coordinate to cause a ripplelike movement that carries intestinal contents along the gut, a process known as *peristalsis*. In the colon the circular muscle may cause segmental contractions that halt the progress of feces or move them back and forth to encourage mixing and metabolic interaction with colon bacteria and mucosa. Gut muscle from the midesophagus to the anus is referred to as

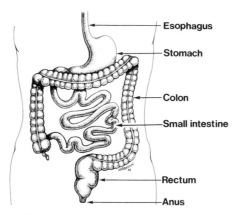

Figure 1-3. The gut. The relationships of the stomach, small intestine, and colon within the abdominal cavity are shown.

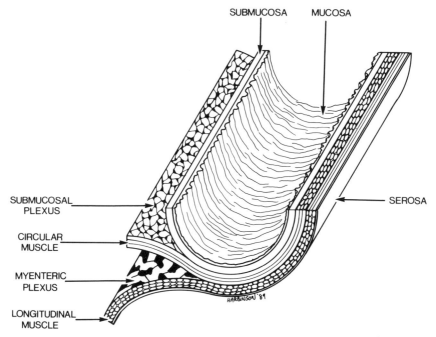

Figure 1-4. The layers of the intestinal wall. Note that the submucosal nerve plexus (network) lies in the submucosa between the mucosa and the circular muscle. The myenteric plexus lies between the two muscle layers. In the small intestine, semicircular folds shown here increase the mucosal surface, maximizing its contact with the intestinal contents.

smooth muscle and is under involuntary control. This distinguishes it from skeletal or *striated* muscle in the limbs (and pharynx and upper esophagus), which is under voluntary control.

The innermost gut layer, the *mucosa*, is also dynamic, although in a metabolic sense. The epithelium is a single layer of cells specialized to handle water, minerals, and nutrients (Figures 1-1 and 1-2). Beneath this cellular layer or *epithelium* the *mucosa* contains a variety of cells that handle absorbed nutrients, or that play a role in the defense against unwanted invaders such as viruses, bacteria, or toxins (see subsequent sections). The mucosa of the colon is diseased in ulcerative colitis, but in Crohn's disease, all three layers are involved at any level of the gut.

The *gastric* (i.e., stomach) mucosa produces a fluid so strongly acidic that it will burn other tissues. For example, you may experience burning in the throat when you vomit. This same acid (hydrochloric) is called muriatic acid by bricklayers, who use it to clean mortar from bricks. The mucosa of the stomach and upper small intestine thus must be metabolically tough enough to resist destruction by the acid and a protein-digesting enzyme called *pepsin*; otherwise, ulceration occurs.

The small-intestinal mucosa is responsible for the absorption of most nutrients, and the daily exchange of about 8 liters of fluid entering the gut from ingestion, or secretion from the intestine, pancreas, and liver. The pancreatic and bile ducts empty pancreatic juice and bile from the pancreas and liver into the upper small intestine. To maximize this enormous fluid exchange, the small-intestinal mucosa is pleated into semicircular folds (Figure 1-4). The epithelial cells are arranged in long fingerlike projections into the lumen called *villi*, which can be seen by microscope (Figure 1-1). To even further increase the gut's luminal surface, each cell has tiny projections called *microvilli*, which are seen only through the electron microscope.

SUPPORT SYSTEMS

Blood Supply

The gut cannot function on its own. It must communicate with the rest of the body for transport of nutrients, gases, and chemical messengers, and for regulation. Three large arteries, the *celiac*, and the *superior* and *inferior mesenteric*, arise from the aorta to supply oxygen and other nutrients to the stomach, small intestine, and colon (the intra-abdominal gut). Corresponding *veins* carry absorbed nutrients and gases away. This process is so efficient that hydrogen gas produced by the action of colon bacteria on ingested intestinal contents appears in the breath within seconds. Tiny vessels called *lymphatics* carry absorbed fats from the small intestine to the circulation.

Nervous System

Gut regulation is effected by the *enteric nervous system* (ENS) and by an ever-increasing list of hormones and *neurotransmitter* substances, which have complex effects on gut movement and fluid transport through the mucosa (Figure 1-4). The ENS is a complex network of nerves and ganglia within the gut wall. The nerve network found between the circular and longitudinal muscle layers is called the *myenteric plexus*. That between the muscle and sub-mucosa is called the *submucous plexus*. Through connections to muscle, mucosa, and blood vessels, this *gut brain* governs our digestion.

The ENS communicates with the brain first via the *sympathetic nerves*, which pass to and from the gut through transformers called *sympathetic ganglia* (Figure 1-5). These nerves connect to the spinal cord, and thence to the base of the brain. Second, *parasympathetic nerves* connect with the base of the brain via the vagus nerve from the upper gut, or the sacral nerves from the colon. Each nerve transmission is affected by one of several neurotransmitters or hormones acting on an appropriate receptor in muscle, nerve ganglion, or other cell. Most of these chemicals are found also in the central nervous system (brain and spinal cord). Some drugs act by mimicking neurotransmitters at their receptors. It is said that the complexity of the ENS or gut brain equals that of the central nervous system, but I would not trust the former to drive a car. From the foregoing one should clearly understand that the brain and the gut are intricately interconnected. Events in the one are unlikely to be ignored by the other!

Protective Mechanisms

The gut is the body's principal port of entry, and its tortuous anatomy constitutes a vast frontier. If the body is to restrict entry, it

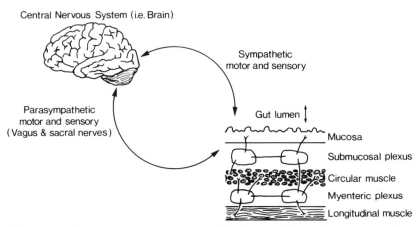

Figure 1-5. The enteric nervous system (ENS). The ENS lies within the gut wall, and through the sympathetic and parasympathetic nerves, transmits and receives information to and from the brain.

must have a customs and immigration service; otherwise, the gut would be subject to invasion not only by nutrients but also by all the microbes, toxins, inert substances, and other flotsam that pass its way. Many protective mechanisms are in place. Gastric acid, bile salts, and pancreatic enzymes conspire to destroy most intestinal contents in the stomach and small bowel. A layer of mucus and a continuous sheet of mucosal epithelial cells lining the lumen of the gut provide a natural barrier (Figures 1-1 and 1-2). The epithelium has great power of repair and can reconstruct itself within hours. Metabolic transport processes carry only nutrients across the barrier. Those items denied entry are carried away by peristalsis. Despite this, invasive bacteria or damaging toxins can breach the epithelial barrier, permitting entrance of unwanted aliens. It thus falls to the body's immune system to police the frontier and destroy or deport the invaders.

Because the immune response is believed to be an important player in the genesis of IBD, a brief description is appropriate here. The gut is very well equipped to mount an immune defense.

Numerous cells in the submucosa and mucosa of the gut possess various immune capabilities (Figures 1-1 and 1-2). Cells with single nuclei, called mononuclear cells, may develop in several directions. Some produce specific antibodies that recognize and attach themselves to foreign proteins, thereby participating in their destruction. Others directly attack the foreigners, some by ingesting them, and others by killing them. The former are called macrophages (literally "big mouth"), and the latter are called killer cells or killer lymphocytes.

The dustup between the immune forces and the invaders results in inflammation. Nearby mast cells release chemical mediators of inflammation, such as histamine, bradykinin, and cytokines. A lipid substance called arachidonic acid is degraded through several steps (regulated by the enzymes cyclooxygenase and lipoxygenase) to produce prostaglandins and leukotrienes. These inflammatory mediators are thought to be important in IBD. Steroids and 5-aminosalicylic acid (5-ASA) compounds used to treat IBD apparently inhibit their production. Blood vessels in the surrounding tissues dilate, causing local congestion with red blood cells (hemorrhage) and fluid (edema). White blood cells called polymorphonuclear cells act as roving policemen in the bloodstream. At the first sign of local trouble, the polymorphs gather at the site—in this case, the gut. These cells have many nuclei, as their name implies, and are important participants in the acute inflammatory response. All of these features may be seen in the mucosa of active ulcerative colitis or in all layers of the gut in Crohn's disease. Whether all this immune activity is in response to some invading foreign substance or microbe yet to be identified, or whether the inflammation results from an intrinsic derangement in the immune system itself, is central to our understanding of the pathogenesis of inflammatory bowel disease (see Chapter 6).

ESOPHAGUS

The esophagus (or gullet) is 20 to 22 centimeters (8 or 9 inches) long and, unlike the intra-abdominal gut, lacks a serosal layer

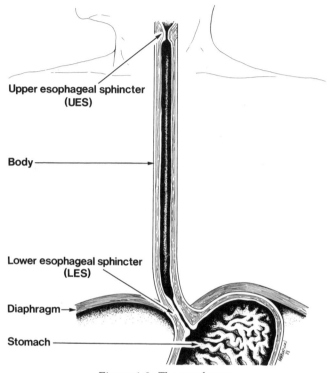

Figure 1-6. The esophagus.

(Figure 1-6). It begins where the pharynx or throat ends, below and behind the Adam's apple. Here the *cricopharyngeous*, a striated muscle under voluntary control, forms the first gut sphincter, called the *upper esophageal sphincter* (UES). This muscular valve must relax before food may be admitted to the gut. The body of the esophagus is powered by striated muscle in its upper third, and smooth muscle in the remainder. More than a passive tube, the esophagus carries food through peristalsis. Thus, the opposum may hang in there without getting up for dinner. At the lower end there is another valve, the *lower esophageal sphincter* (LES), which must relax as food arrives, yet normally maintains a pressure that prevents gastric contents from refluxing into the esophagus. The LES is normally at the diaphragm where the gut enters the abdomen.

STOMACH

The stomach is a nice organ to take to the dinner table.
Lester Dragstedt

It is curious that an organ about which so much has been written is not essential for life. With altered eating habits, nutritional care, and vitamin B_{12} injections, patients whose stomachs have been surgically removed may live for many years. Nonetheless, the stomach stores and mixes a meal, begins the digestive process, and is the putative source of many digestive complaints.

The stomach is a variably shaped organ resembling a fat reclining "J" (Figure 1-7). It has three parts: the *cardia* lying above the *fundus*; the fundus or *body*, which extends from the cardia vertically

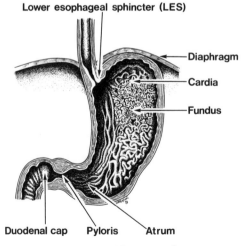

Figure 1-7. The stomach.

downward; and the *antrum*, which is the foot of the "J," ending at a thickened muscular ring called the *pylorus*. The upper stomach is a container, whereas the antrum has mixing and pumping actions. The circular muscle layer of the stomach is separated from that of the duodenum by the pylorus, the third valve or sphincter that we encounter as we travel down the gut.

SMALL INTESTINE

The small intestine (Figure 1-8) plays the major role in absorption of nutrients. It is attached to the posterior wall of the abdomen by the *mesentery*, a ligament that contains the blood vessels, nerves, and lymphatics. There are three segments within the small intestine: the *duodenum*, the *jejunum*, and the *ileum*. The first part of the duodenum, that just beyond the pylorus, is called the duodenal cap. It is here that duodenal ulcers usually occur. The remainder of the duodenum encircles the head of the pancreas and ends at a sharp angulation called the *ligament of Treitz* (Figure 1-8). The *common bile duct* and *pancreatic ducts* originate in the liver and pancreas, respectively, and enter the duodenum at the *ampulla of Vater*.

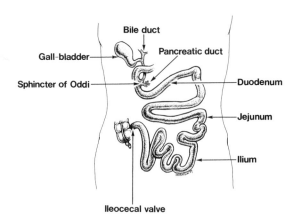

Figure 1-8. The small intestine. The duodenum becomes the jejunum at the ligament of Treitz, a sharp angulation of the gut near the splenic flexure of colon. Note that both pancreatic juice, which contains digestive enzymes, and bile, which contains bile salts, enter the duodenum through the sphincter of Oddi.

The *jejunum* is the longest segment and is the most important in terms of absorption of water, minerals, and nutrients. No feature marks the imperceptible junction of the jejunum with the *ileum*. The ileum is the site of absorption of vitamin B_{12} and bile salts, and terminates at the next gut sphincter, the *ileocecal valve*.

THE COLON

The Flanders of medicine
Spriggs, 1930

Another organ we can apparently do without, the colon is nonetheless the site of many gut miseries. In Figure 1-9 one should note that the colon or large intestine begins at the ileocecal valve with the cecum and ascending colon. This organ travels up the right side of the abdomen, turning at the hepatic flexure to cross the upper abdomen as the transverse colon, and then at the splenic flexure, it descends down the left side to the sigmoid colon and rectum. It is well to recognize at this point that our colons contain myriad bacteria with which we have great interdependence. The

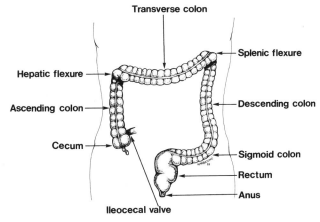

Figure 1-9. The colon.

digestive process is completed in the cecum and right side of the colon by these intestinal bacteria. As much as a liter of water is reabsorbed by the colon, and a semisolid fecal mass remains. The *rectum* acts as a storage container.

THE ANORECTUM

The storage and evacuation of feces and the maintenance of continence are complex and will be discussed in Chapter 2. The rectum (Figure 1-10) is a spacious organ lying in front of the sacrum and behind the vagina and bladder. Several anatomical features serve to hold back feces in the rectum. These include the sharp anorectal angle, which is maintained by the *puborectalis*, a pelvic floor muscle shown in the diagram. A series of semilunar projections into the lower rectum, called *rectal valves*, check the fecal flow. Finally, there are two *anal sphincters*. The inner one consists of smooth muscle and is under ENS control. The external anal sphincter consists of striated or voluntary muscle, and one learns to control it through toilet training.

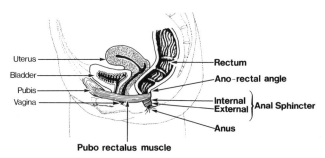

Figure 1-10. The Anorectum. The semilunar rectal valves help slow the fecal flow. When rectal distention with stool stimulates the defecation reflex, the puborectalis muscle relaxes, straightening the anorectal angle. The internal anal sphincter relaxes, and the descending colon contracts. Defecation is prevented if one voluntarily contracts the external anal sphincter.

PERITONEUM

Most of the abdominal gut is coiled within a potential space called the *peritoneal* space. The peritoneal surface of the gut is lined by a thin layer of cells called the serosa (see the preceding). This serosal layer is continuous with the peritoneum, which becomes a large convoluted envelope. When an inflamed gut perforates, gut contents soil the normally sterile peritoneal space. If the space is walled off by inflammatory tissue, as in Crohn's disease, a local abscess occurs. If not, as in a perforated toxic megacolon, generalized peritonitis occurs, which is a grave surgical emergency.

SUMMARY

The gut is a 9-meter-long muscular organ commencing at the throat and ending at the anus. There is an outer longitudinal muscle layer and an inner circular muscle layer. The coordinated contractions (peristalsis) of these layers move intestinal contents in a manner programmed by the ENS in the gut wall, which is in turn influenced by neurotransmitters, hormones, and connections to the central nervous system. The mucosa lines the gut lumen and is responsible for the absorption of nutrients and secretion of acid and enzymes. It is also under ENS control. Numerous natural barriers and a profound immune capability guard the gut frontier against invasion by microorganisms and toxins. The esophagus is an active muscular conduit with upper and lower esophageal sphincters. The upper stomach acts as a meal container where acid and pepsin are secreted and digestion begins. The lower stomach, the antrum, is a pump that grinds food and injects measured amounts of gastric contents through the pylorus into the upper intestine. The jejunum and ileum of the small intestine serve to absorb nutrients, and the ileum terminates in the ileocecal valve. The colon is a bacteria-filled organ that changes semifluid small-intestinal contents into feces. The anatomic configuration of the rectum and anus is vital to normal defecation and continence.

CHAPTER TWO

How the Gut Works

A *mouthful*, once swallowed, becomes a *bolus*, which is carried to the stomach where it is mixed and partly digested into *chyme*. On entering the upper small bowel, it becomes *intestinal contents*, which are altered by absorption and secretion through the intestinal mucosa. Somewhere farther down, the intestinal contents become known as *feces* or *stool*, certainly in the lower colon and beyond. In order that these metamorphoses may occur in an orderly fashion, gut smooth muscle must convey luminal contents in a manner consistent with optimal digestion. This process is governed by the enteric nervous system (ENS) and its neurotransmitters, which in turn are influenced by hormones and interconnections with the brain. The motility of the gut is influenced by a variety of reflexes, which respond to the concentration, osmolarity, size, and nature of the luminal contents and to events occurring elsewhere in the gut. Thus, when in perfect harmony, various segments of the gut accept food and move it along, extracting the water, salts, and nutrients needed by the body. Ultimately a soft, formed, easily passed stool is prepared to be evacuated from the rectum at a time convenient to its owner. Normally, all this occurs without entering consciousness. This chapter discusses the manner in which the gut works, that is, its physiology.

THE ESOPHAGUS (GULLET)

The upper esophageal sphincter (UES) is the first one-way valve that the food bolus encounters as it begins its journey down the gullet. (The mouth might be considered to be the first by some, but it is neither one way, nor involuntary.) When food is swallowed, the UES must relax to allow it to pass into the esophagus. This valve may help prevent food and gastric juice that escapes from the stomach into the esophagus from refluxing into the throat.

The body of the esophagus is not a simple conduit. Its inner and outer muscular layers coordinate to produce primary peristalsis: a wave of increased intraesophageal pressure preceded by relaxation. This wave normally carries a bolus of food before it into the stomach, a process that takes approximately 7 seconds. With age, peristalsis may occur with only 50 percent of swallows, and there may be nonperistaltic (tertiary) contractions. Distention of the esophagus initiates *secondary peristalsis*, an important mechanism for clearing the esophagus of food or acid refluxed from the stomach. Impaired clearing of acid from the body of the esophagus may contribute to heartburn.

Anatomists have failed to identify any thickening of the muscle layer that they could call the *lower esophageal sphincter* (LES). Electronic sensors that record intraluminal pressure, however, do detect a high-pressure zone about 3 centimeters long just above the point where the esophagus empties into the stomach [the *gastroesophageal (GE) junction*]. In response to the arrival of a peristaltic wave, this one-way valve relaxes to allow the esophageal contents to be discharged into the stomach. Normally LES pressure, as measured by intraluminal sensors, is greater than the intraluminal pressure of the stomach. When part of the stomach herniates (protrudes) through the diaphragm up into the chest, one has a *hiatus hernia*. Hiatus hernia and heartburn are both very common and must commonly occur together by coincidence. Nevertheless, anatomic relationships are of some importance. The sharp angle (angle of Hiss) at which the esophagus enters the stomach may serve as a flutter valve. The normal intra-abdominal location of the LES just below the diaphragm may help prevent it from being overwhelmed by increases in abdominal pressure.

STOMACH

Gastric Motility

As a storage container, the stomach expands to accommodate a meal with little change in intragastric pressure. Such fine adjustment of gastric capacity is regulated by tonic contractions and relaxations. *Volume* or *capacity* contractions last about a minute and involve primarily the proximal (upper) stomach. They control gastric emptying of liquids but not of solids.

Gastric peristaltic waves begin at midstomach and spread as a circumferential band through the antrum to the pylorus. They are of two types: the first is smaller weak waves, which have a mixing function, and the second is larger more powerful waves, which have a propulsive as well as a mixing action. After a meal, conditions are such that each electrical slow wave may initiate a peristaltic contraction; these occur at the rate of three per minute. The stomach selectively empties liquids while retaining solids larger than 2 millimeters in size. This capacity depends on the antrum and pylorus acting in concert. The pylorus can be seen radiographically and endoscopically to open and close. Antral contractions regularly propel gastric contents toward the pylorus, through which small amounts are squirted into the duodenum. Most contents, including larger particles that are unable to pass the pylorus, are retropelled into the proximal stomach through the nozzle formed by the advancing peristaltic wave. In this fashion, the meal is mixed and ground into particles small enough to be acted on by the intestine.

In contrast to the postmeal state, the fasting stomach undergoes a three-phase cycle: inactive; irregular contractions; and a terminal intense peristaltic phase that sweeps all before it into the duodenum. This cycle may take 1 to 2 hours. The stomach thus is a receptacle, a mixer, and a grinder. The pylorus is the gatekeeper of the intestine, controlling the rate and form in which food is presented for digestion. Gastric function is subject to many external influences, the composition of its contents, and the activity of the ENS.

SMALL INTESTINE

"Local stimulation of the gut produces excitation above and inhibition below the excited spot." This is the law of the intestine, expounded by the pioneering physiologists Bayliss and Starling in 1899. Spontaneous small-bowel motility is more complex, and cannot be dealt with in detail here. Basically, there are nonpropulsive and propulsive contractions. The former are discoordinated and occur at adjacent sites in the intestine. These move the gut contents back and forth in pendulum fashion. The contractions are most active following a meal and serve to mix the intestinal contents and ensure maximal contact with the absorbing surface of the mucosa.

In the period between meals there are cycles of propagating contractions lasting from 2 to 2.5 hours. These are the *migrating motor complexes* (MMC), which correspond to small-intestinal peristalsis. This peristalsis is characterized by a moving ring, formed by circular muscle contraction, preceded by relaxation. The role of the MMCs and peristalsis is to keep the normally sterile small gut clear of residual food and help limit bacteria. In addition, there are infrequent powerful or giant migrating contractions that originate in the distal small bowel and sweep through the colon into the rectum. They precede defecation and correspond to the colon "mass movements" described by radiologists. These peristaltic rushes of barium were vividly described early in this century by the American physiologist, Cannon. Segmentation and peristalsis are functions of the circular muscle coat, whereas volume control and a sleeving action of the gut are functions of the longitudinal layer. Reverse peristalsis probably does not normally occur, because electrical impulses are transmitted only toward the rectum. Abnormalities of small-intestinal contractions may be responsible for symptoms. Migrating motor complexes may be more frequent and cover a greater length of gut in diarrhea. Spontaneous giant migrating ileal contractions appear to coincide with cramps.

There is a remarkable exchange of fluids, minerals, and nutrients across the mucosa. It is estimated that the small intestine handles as much as 8 liters of fluid from ingestion and from secretion by stomach, intestine, liver, and pancreas. In cholera, absorption by the small intestine is blocked by the cholera toxin, and the result is severe diarrhea, dehydration and, if untreated, death. Small alterations in this extensive fluid exchange could play a role in constipation or diarrhea. Generally speaking, laxatives increase net small-bowel secretion, whereas antidiarrheal agents decrease it.

The motor, absorptive, and secretory functions of the small intestine may be profoundly altered in a segment afflicted with Crohn's disease. Relative obstruction in such a segment may cause strong contractions above (cramps) and loss of fluid into the dilated gut lumen.

COLON

Our digestions . . . going sacredly and silently right, that is the foundation of all poetry . . . the most poetical thing in the world is not being sick.

C. K. Chesterton (1908)

During passage of the intestinal contents from the ileum through the colon, about a liter of fluid is absorbed, and semisolid feces are presented to the rectum. In perfusion studies, as much as 7 liters may be absorbed in 24 hours, but much less if the fluid is presented in boluses, such as after meals. The fluid salvage operation is impaired when the colon mucosa is inflamed; in colitis, this impairment is the principal determinant of diarrhea. Colon bacteria alter the solid portion by digestion of nonabsorbed glycoproteins and carbohydrates such as cellulose. The gases hydrogen, carbon dioxide, and methane are produced, along with volatile fatty acids, which have both cathartic and nutritive function. These are absorbed or expelled, and the final fecal mass is largely water with the major solid component consisting of bacteria.

Early in the twentieth century before the dangers of x-rays were known, a succession of distinguished investigators observed the passage of radiopaque material through the colon. From their work and the recent use of intracolonic pressure-sensing devices, a concept of colon motility has emerged. There are three modes of colon motor activity. The first is basic tone, superimposed upon which are the second, nonpropulsive, segmenting contractions. The third is the mass propulsive activity discussed under the small intestine. The dominant colon movement is nonpropulsive segmentation, which is most vigorous in the descending colon and sigmoid. These contractions may occur randomly or may be coordinated, but their propulsive activity is small.

Radiologically observed mass movements in the colon occur in response to an unknown force. Because they are infrequent, they are difficult to study. Unlike true peristalsis seen in the small bowel, a mass movement is apparently not caused by a migrating contraction ring preceded by relaxation. After a segment of colon has kneaded the feces for several hours, segmental contractions disappear, and the bolus is mysteriously advanced. In colitis, control of these movements is lost, further contributing to diarrhea.

Mental and physical stress alter colon contractions, and a meal, especially fat, may stimulate the colon. Thus, the central nervous system, the ENS and hormones play important roles in colon regulation. The mechanisms that tune colon secretion, absorption, propulsion, retropulsion, and segmentation are intricate indeed and may be profoundly disturbed when the gut is inflamed or scarred. Chesterton is correct. Our digestions "going sacredly and silently right" *are* poetic.

DEFECATION

The rectum is normally empty. Perhaps because of awareness of a full colon or perhaps in response to eating, the descending colon and sigmoid straighten, and undergo an integrated contraction that delivers feces into the rectum. Tonic contraction of the internal anal sphincter maintains continence (Figure 1-10). Rectal distention reflexly relaxes the internal sphincter and contracts the external sphincter. Continence is then maintained by the external sphincter until one is ready for voluntary defecation. Upright posture and increased intra-abdominal pressure also cause the external sphincter to contract. The rectum can accommodate 100 to 200 grams before the defecation reflex is initiated.

With defecation the puborectalis muscle relaxes and descends, removing the 80- to 100-degree anorectal angle. The external sphincter relaxes, and the descending colon contracts, pushing the feces through the now funnel-shaped and patent anus. This should completely empty the left colon, which appears to function independent of the right. This activity is accompanied to a variable extent by abdominal muscle contraction, diaphragm descent, and forced expiration against a closed glottis (straining).

Continence is a uniquely human attribute. To be sure, there are primeval reflexes that prevent accidental defecation as a consequence of temporary increases in abdominal pressure, but the voluntary retention of feces through the third act of *Aida* is a phenomenon unique to civilized man. To this end there are two factors of vital importance. The first is conscious control over the voluntary muscles of the external sphincter and pelvic floor. Voluntary closure of the external sphincter and contraction of the puborectalis muscle to sharpen the anorectal angle makes the anal canal a narrow slit. The cushionlike hemorrhoidal veins are squeezed together by the sphincter and act as a seal against increases in intra-abdominal pressure. The second continence factor is the very rich sensory innervation of the anal canal within and above the anal sphincter, which allows the individual to distinguish feces from fluids or flatus. When rectal distention relaxes the internal sphincter, it exposes the sensitive anal mucosa to intestinal content; thus, one may decide whether to drop one's drink and run, or to close the external sphincter, tighten up the puborectalis, and finish that fascinating conversation. Habitual adoption of the latter course could lead to constipation.

A number of physiologic abnormalities may produce symptoms in inflammatory bowel disease (IBD). In advanced ulcerative colitis, the colon and rectum become a rigid, narrowed tube. Uncontrolled, feces sluice into the rectum, which has reduced storage and absorption capacity. The result is frequent, urgent, watery defecation to the point of incontinence, even when the inflammation is not active. Damage to the puborectalis muscle and internal sphincter may contribute to constipation, as may weak colorectal contractions or lack of sensation of a full rectum. Incontinence may result from decreased perception of watery stool in the rectum, increased stool volume, loss of the mucosal plug after anal surgery, loss of the anorectal angle, decreased sphincter pressure, or damage to the sphincter and pelvic floor. Such damage or destruction may result from Crohn's disease. The resulting fissures, fistulas, abscesses, disturbed defecation, and incontinence are the most frustrating and damaging features of this chronic, young people's disease.

SUMMARY

From the stomach, distally, the timing of gut smooth muscle contractions is determined by rhythmic electrical activity. Contractions seem to be influenced by the ENS, subject to activity in the central nervous system and to hormones.

In response to a swallow, the UES relaxes, allowing passage of the bolus into the esophageal body, down the length of which it is carried by peristalsis. The LES relaxes with the arrival of the food bolus, thus allowing the peristaltic wave to sweep all before it into the stomach. Impaired tone of the LES or incomplete peristalsis may permit acid, pepsin, and sometimes bile to reflux into the esophagus, causing heartburn and in some cases esophagitis.

The body of the stomach adjusts the gastric capacity for food by means of tonic contractions and relaxations. Gastric peristalsis begins in midbody and may sweep through into the duodenum or may terminate in a vigorous contraction against a closed pylorus that helps to mix and grind the food. The antrum and pylorus, acting in concert, prevent the reflux of duodenal contents into the stomach. Inflammatory bowel disease may disrupt these functions through local disease, obstruction lower down, or drug side-effects.

In the small gut, a series of contractions occurs 4 or 5 centimeters apart, dividing intraluminal contents into segments, mixing the contents, and maximizing mucosal exposure. The migrating motor complex (peristalsis) consists of a moving contraction ring that travels only a few centimeters.

Nonpropulsive segmentation is more common in the left colon than in the right. It mixes and slows the progress of colon contents. Mass movements or peristalsis are rarely recognized. A normal bowel movement is thus a balance of these mechanical forces and the amount of fluid presented to and absorbed from the colon. Lack of coordination and mucosal inflammation cause the abdominal pain, diarrhea, constipation, and other symptoms found in IBD.

Defecation is initiated when contraction of the right colon delivers feces into the rectum. Rectal distension relaxes the internal anal sphincter, but continence can be voluntarily maintained by the external sphincter, which squeezes shut the anal mucosa and hemorrhoidal venous cushions. With defecation, the pelvic floor (puborectalis) relaxes and descends, removing the sharp angle between the anus and the rectum. The descending colon contracts, delivering feces through the funnel-shaped and patent anus.

CHAPTER THREE

Nosology and Nomenclature

The ill and unfit choice of words wonderfully obstructs the understanding.

Francis Bacon (1561–1626)

Don't sir, accustom yourself to use big words for little matters . . . The
practice of using words of disproportionate magnitude is, no doubt, too
frequent.

Samuel Johnson (1709–1784)

A nosologist is not one who knows everything, or a specialist in
noses, but rather one who classifies diseases. The nosology of
inflammatory bowel disease (IBD) is based on two distinct pathologic processes, ulcerative colitis and Crohn's disease (regional
ileitis), subdivided into their respective anatomical predilections in
the gut (Table 3-1). This chapter enunciates this classification and
defines some of the terminology associated with it. Those giants of
English literature, Bacon and Johnson, give good advice. Unfortunately, medical terminology is a mixture of many languages, both
ancient and modern, and the result is often obfuscation rather than
clarification. Nevertheless, terms such as *dysplasia*, *proctosigmoiditis*,
and even *stricturoplasty* are commonly employed in discussions of
IBD, and we must respect them here.

TABLE 3-1
Inflammatory Bowel Disease

Ulcerative colitis
  Proctitis
  Proctosigmoiditis
  Left-sided colitis
  Pancolitis
Crohn's disease
  Crohn's colitis
  Ileocecal Crohn's
  Small-bowel Crohn's
  Other (esophagus, stomach, duodenum, etc.)
Indeterminate colitis

INFLAMMATORY BOWEL DISEASE

The term *IBD* the topic of this book, is very imprecise. Theoretically, it could refer to any inflammatory condition of the bowel. This would include not only enteric infections by microorganisms such as shigella or ameba, but also such common afflictions as appendicitis or diverticulitis. More rarely, inflammation of the bowel due to a foreign body might be embraced by the term. But usage has firmly established IBD as the generic term for ulcerative colitis and Crohn's disease, and it assumes the absence of other inflammatory conditions of the bowel. Nevertheless, many of these other inflammatory conditions may be confused with the acute stages of ulcerative colitis or Crohn's disease. Usually, the confusion is short lived. Infections are acute and quickly over, whereas IBD is chronic and recurring. Whether ulcerative colitis and regional enteritis are distinct from one another is the subject of much speculation. In our discussions, we consider them separately.

ULCERATIVE COLITIS

Ulcerative colitis is an inflammation confined to the mucosa, or inner lining, of the colon. It almost always begins at the anorectum and extends to a variable degree proximally (toward the cecum). This variability in disease extent gives rise to the subclassification discussed subsequently. Rarely is the anorectum spared in ulcerative colitis, and if so, one should consider the possibility of Crohn's disease.

Ulcerative Proctitis

Proctitis is from the Greek word meaning anus or rectum. In ulcerative proctitis (Figure 3-1), the features of ulcerative colitis are confined to the anorectum. This condition usually follows a chronic, relapsing course, similar to that of ulcerative colitis. Unlike colitis, however, there are seldom systemic features such as weight loss, fever, or anemia. In about 10 percent of cases of ulcerative proctitis, the disease may spread more proximally, that is, toward the cecum.

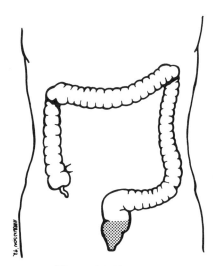

Figure 3-1. Proctitis.

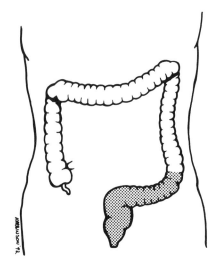

Figure 3-2. Proctosigmoiditis.

Proctosigmoiditis

Sigmoid, another word of Greek derivation, means S-shaped. Proctosigmoiditis (Figure 3-2) extends beyond the rectum into the sigmoid or S-shaped colon. The severity of the disease tends to vary with its extent. Proctosigmoiditis sufferers are thus usually more troubled than those with proctitis, and systemic features may be present.

Left-Sided Colitis

Another step up the severity scale, left-sided colitis (Figure 3-3) extends from the anus proximally to near the splenic flexure or to the transverse colon. All the complications of ulcerative colitis may be seen with this variant.

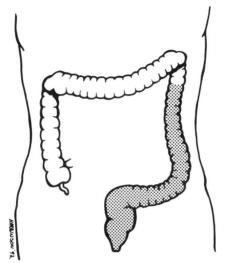

Figure 3-3. Left-sided colitis.

Pancolitis

In some cases of colitis (Figure 3-4), the whole colon is involved. This is known as pancolitis. Sufferers of pancolitis are usually the most severely ill, and most subject to the serious complications of ulcerative colitis, such as cancer, major hemorrhage, or toxic mega-colon.

CROHN'S DISEASE (REGIONAL ENTERITIS)

The terms *Crohn's disease* and *regional enteritis* are used inter-changeably. The latter more precisely describes the disease, but the former has the advantage of widespread use. Unlike those in ulcerative colitis, all three layers of the gut are involved in Crohn's disease—the mucosa, the muscular layer, and the outer serosal coat. The disease may be found from mouth to anus, but most commonly in the large and small intestine. Uniquely, areas of normal gut called *skip areas* may be found between two affected segments. Occa-

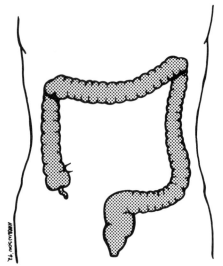

Figure 3-4. Pancolitis.

sionally the lesions of Crohn's disease may be found remote from the gut, such as in the skin, larynx, and bladder.

Crohn's Colitis

The whole colon or any part of it may be involved with Crohn's disease (Figure 3-5). Unlike that in ulcerative colitis, the rectum may be spared, and more than one segment may be involved. The term *granulomatous colitis* may be used. Granulomas are occasional histologic features of Crohn's not usually found in ulcerative colitis. In some cases the small bowel is involved as well. Because it is very common today, it is surprising that Crohn's disease was not generally thought to involve the colon prior to 1960.

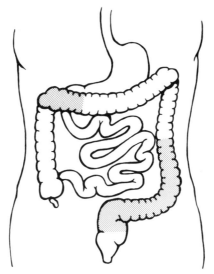

Figure 3-5. Crohn's colitis. Note rectal sparing and skip areas.

Ileocecal Crohn's

Early reports of Crohn's disease described inflammation of the terminal ileum, and Crohn and his associates suggested the term *terminal ileitis*. We now recognize that the cecum is very frequently involved as well. Ileocecal Crohn's (Figure 3-6) is the most common Crohn's variant.

Small-Bowel Crohn's Disease

In this case, the disease is usually confined to the small bowel, and the terminal ileum may be spared. A less common variant, small-bowel Crohn's (Figure 3-7) is responsible for the most serious nutritional problems of IBD. Sometimes the term *jejunoileitis* is used.

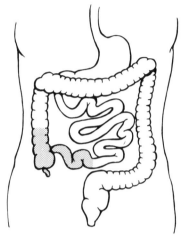

Figure 3-6. Ileocecal Crohn's.

Other

Any segment of the gut may be involved in Crohn's disease. The subgroup of Crohn's is indicated by the anatomic site, as in Crohn's disease of the duodenum, or esophagus. Perianal Crohn's signifies disease about the anus, usually manifest as fissures, fistulas, or local sepsis.

INDETERMINATE COLITIS

In as many as 10 percent of colonic IBD cases, it is initially impossible to determine whether ulcerative colitis or Crohn's is present. It may take many months or even years for the disease to declare itself. A case initially diagnosed as ulcerative colitis with the typical sigmoidoscopic and radiologic features may later be revealed to be regional enteritis through the discovery of skip areas or small-bowel involvement, or through examination of the whole gut wall at

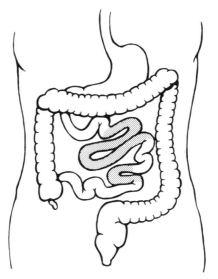

Figure 3-7. Small-bowel Crohn's.

surgery. On the other hand, initial presentation of Crohn's disease that turns out to be ulcerative colitis seems rare. Occasionally, ulcerative colitis may at first be confined to the right colon. If the colonoscopic, radiologic, and histologic features favor colitis, the term *right-sided colitis* may be used, with the full realization that it may yet be Crohn's.

COMPLICATIONS

Ulcerative Colitis Complications

There are many local and systemic complications of ulcerative colitis. These will be discussed in detail later, but a few new terms should be introduced now. *Fulminant colitis* is a life-threatening severe attack of the disease, with a very ill, toxic patient. *Toxic megacolon* is the late state of severe, acute disease in which the colon becomes stretched, dilated, thinned, and perforation threatens. This situation provokes emergency removal of the colon (colectomy).

Dysplasia is a histologic change in the colon mucosa in chronic ulcerative colitis, and is considered a harbinger of colon carcinoma (see Chapter 17). *Backwash ileitis* is a benign inflammation of the terminal ileum, which is found in cases of pancolitis.

Crohn's Disease Complications

All layers of the gut are involved in Crohn's disease. This feature accounts for its most serious complications. Destruction of the gut wall may result in a *fistula*, that is, a track or fault in the wall of the intestine permitting the contents to escape. Such fistulas may result in free perforation into the peritoneum, an abscess adjacent to the gut, or penetration into the muscles of the pelvic floor. Fistulas may track into other organs, such as the skin (enterocutaneous), vagina (enterovaginal), bladder (enterovesicle), gut (enteroenteral), or perineum (perianal). Especially in the small gut, narrowing or obstruction may occur because of inflammation in the wall. If the narrowing is due to scarring, it is irreversible and is called a *stricture*.

EXTRAINTESTINAL MANIFESTATIONS

As many as 100 conditions associated with IBD occur in organs remote from the gut. These include such diverse diseases as *sclerosing cholangitis* (bile ducts), *erythema nodosum* and *pyoderma gangrenosum* (skin), *rheumatoid spondylitis* (spine), and *iritis* (eye) (see Chapter 16).

SURGICAL GLOSSARY

A *colectomy* is the surgical removal of the colon. In a total colectomy, the organ from cecum to anus is removed, whereas a subtotal colectomy spares the rectum. The former is the operation generally done for ulcerative colitis, whereas the latter, lesser operation may be done in a very ill patient with colitis, or colonic Crohn's disease. *Proctectomy* means removal of the rectum, and a total colectomy is sometimes known as a *proctocolectomy*. An ileal resection implies removal of part of the ileum, and is done usually for Crohn's disease. The ileocecal valve and part of the ascending colon are usually removed as well. Resections of other segments of the large or small bowel may be done for Crohn's disease. *Stricturoplasty* is a local attempt to repair a small-bowel stricture without removing bowel.

An *ileostomy* is the insertion of the cut end of the ileum into the abdominal wall as an outlet for intestinal contents after the colon has been removed. When the colon is brought to light in the same manner, the result is called a *colostomy*. This is necessary when the rectum is removed or severely affected with Crohn's disease. The site of such a bowel extrusion is called a *stoma* or *ostomy*. A *loop ostomy* is a temporary connection of a bowel loop to the skin as a diverting or decompressing device. The site where two segments of bowel are joined after a resection is called an *anastomosis* (e.g., ileocecal anastomosis). This is a frequent site for Crohn's disease recurrence.

CHAPTER FOUR

History of Inflammatory Bowel Disease

Ulcerative colitis and regional enteritis are diseases of the twentieth century. Almost all that we know about them has been learned in the last 80 years. It is impossible to imagine, however, that these diseases did not exist previously. Case descriptions dating to antiquity, which some medical historians believe are of inflammatory bowel disease (IBD), have been flushed from the writings of Aretaeus the Cappadocian (born in 80 AD), Sydenham in 1666, Morgagni in 1767, and Cruveilhier (born in 1791). It is impossible to verify such claims, because the authors had primitive notions of pathology, and no notion at all of infectious diseases that even today may mimic IBD.

During the nineteenth century, descriptions of disease became more articulate, and putative IBD cases became more credible and numerous. The most celebrated case was that of a Miss Bankes, whose 1859 autopsy description by Wilkes was considered the first bona fide case of ulcerative colitis. It seems that she was married to a certain Doctor Swethurst of London, who was charged with her murder by poisoning. Testimony by Wilkes and the defendant's other wife, Mary, resulted in dismissal of the murder charge and the laying of a new charge of bigamy. Ironically, Fielding recently reviewed the case and, noting colon and small-bowel involvement, judged that, after all, Miss Bankes was afflicted with Crohn's disease. The truth about Miss Bankes may still be unfolding.

ULCERATIVE COLITIS

In the late eighteenth century, the works of Koch, Pasteur, and Lister led to awareness of infectious agents as specific causes of diseases. Enteric infections became known as well. In 1875, Wilkes and Moxon were able to confidently describe cases of noninfectious inflammation of the large intestine as *idiopathic colitis*, that is, colitis of unknown cause. In the 1880s and 90s, Italian and British surgeons began cautiously to perform colostomies for this affliction, and the first authentic descriptions of the pathology of ulcerative colitis were written.

The first systematic descriptions of the clinical findings, treatment, and statistical data of ulcerative colitis were presented at the Royal Society of Medicine, London, in 1909. Many European and American reports followed. Although blood transfusions introduced in the 1920s improved many patients, most contemporary treatments were dubious, and had no basis in science or systematic experience. They reflected ancient folk traditions and ignorance of pathogenesis rather than rational and tested approaches. In the 1930s, colitis was considered a psychosomatic disease, and psychiatric therapy dominated.

The first significant advance in the treatment of ulcerative colitis was the introduction of sulfasalazine by Nana Svartz in 1940. Svartz, a Swedish physician, first tested the drug in the treatment of rheumatoid arthritis. Some of her patients, who also had ulcerative colitis, noticed improvement in their gut symptoms, and subsequent trials proved the efficacy of the drug in mild to moderate disease. Interestingly this drug is enjoying a modest revival as a treatment for rheumatoid arthritis. In 1952, Truelove and Witts of Oxford introduced adrenocorticotropin and corticosteroids for the treatment of ulcerative colitis. For many years after that, a debate raged over the relative merits of these two drugs. The former, a pituitary hormone that stimulates the release of corticosteroids from the adrenal glands, is seldom used now.

CROHN'S DISEASE (REGIONAL ENTERITIS)

Beginning with Morgagni in 1776, and throughout the nineteenth century, there appeared many clinical descriptions compatible with regional enteritis. These descriptions are redolent of Victorian imagery; thus, the lumen of the narrowed intestine is "the size of a turkey quill" or a "swan's quill." Also, "The affected bowel gives the consistence and smoothness of an eel in a state of rigor mortis" (Dalziel, 1913).

It is an accident of history that the eponym *Crohn* became attached to regional enteritis. Not only did many case reports precede the famous report of Crohn, Ginsberg, and Oppenheimer, but a Glasgow surgeon, T. K. Dalziel, also reported 13 cases in the *British Medical Journal* in 1913. Had his report not been followed by his death and the distraction of World War I, the condition might well be known as Dalziel's disease. Certainly much of his clinical and pathological account of the disease is valid today; Crohn's coauthors might equally claim immortality, but the authors were named alphabetically.

Nevertheless, it was the 1932 paper by Crohn and his colleagues in the *Journal of the American Medical Association* that led to widespread recognition of the disease. Oddly, all 14 patients reported in that study had disease of the terminal ileum, and terminal ileitis was the suggested descriptor. When the paper was presented in New Orleans in 1932, Bargen from the Mayo Clinic suggested the name *regional enteritis*, thus anticipating recognition of the variable location of the disease in the small and large bowel. Although colon involvement with regional enteritis was reported in the 1950s (indeed Wilkes' 1859 case involved the colon), it was not until reports from London and Oxford in 1960 that Crohn's disease of the colon was established as a valid entity.

Because Dalziel missed immortality by happenstance, he might be permitted to have the last word in this section. His 1913 optimism seems misplaced even now.

> I can only regret that the etiology of the condition remains in obscurity, but I trust that ere long further consideration will clear up the difficulty.

OTHER IBD LANDMARKS

In 1895, Hale-White reported an association of ulcerative colitis with liver disease, the first of a long list of extraintestinal manifestations of IBD. Lockhart-Mummery in 1907 described seven instances of colon carcinoma among 36 patients with ulcerative colitis, thus identifying ulcerative colitis as a pre-cancerous disease. The same author pointed out the importance of the sigmoidoscope in the diagnosis and monitoring of the disease at the Royal Society of Medicine meeting in 1909. At that same conference, the familial nature of ulcerative colitis was described.

Through the 1930s, work at the Mayo and Lahey clinics provided information about the chronic relapsing course of ulcerative colitis and the potentially deadly consequences of massive hemorrhage and toxic dilatation. Growth retardation was recognized in adolescents afflicted with the disease. Sclerosing cholangitis became known as the most important liver complication. Although ulcerative colitis seemed to be the dominant IBD into the 1940s, by 1960 Crohn's disease was almost equally prevalent. The latter disease is at least as common now.

Colectomy became a cure for ulcerative colitis, and in the 1930s, Crohn's disease too was considered a surgical disease. Attempts to extirpate all the affected intestine, after the cancer model, led to short bowels and much surgical morbidity. Recurrences at the anastomotic site encouraged even more aggressive resections. The minimalist view of surgical treatment of Crohn's disease is a relatively recent phenomenon.

THE MODERN VIEW

We are little wiser about the cause of IBD than was Dalziel in 1913, but there seems to be a derangement of the immune response, either as a primary event, or as an overresponse to an as-yet-unidentified antigen. The clinical manifestations of the two diseases have been recorded in great detail. Nearly 100 extraintestinal manifestations of IBD have been catalogued. The Crohn's Disease Activity Index (CDAI), developed as a part of the U.S. National Cooperative Crohn's Disease Study in 1979, represents the first attempt to quantitate the activity of the disease from period to period (Chapter 24). The index proved cumbersome for regular use, and simplifications are still being proposed. The point is that there is a recognized need to measure the course of the disease if therapies are to be evaluated. The systematic assessment of psychosocial factors and quality of life is a recent innovation (see Chapter 18).

Medical treatment has developed principally from the empirical discoveries of Svartz and Truelove. Sulfasalazine consists of 5-aminosalicylic (5-ASA) bound to sulfapyridine. Because sulfasalazine has been recognized as a delivery system for 5-ASA, and the sulfonamide part of the molecule is the cause of most side-effects, why not simply give 5-ASA? A recent flurry of pharmaceutical activity has brought forth several new delivery systems for 5-ASA (see Chapter 20). Cortisone has been replaced by systemic and topical corticosteroids with fewer undesired effects (Chapter 21). New trials may lead to the release of nonabsorbable steroids or steroids rapidly metabolized in the liver. Azathioprine, an immunosuppressant drug, was shown in the 1979 National Cooperative Crohn's Disease Study to permit patients to control their disease with smaller doses of prednisone. A closely related drug, 6-mercaptopurine, seemed to be validated by a small study in 1980, but immunosuppressants are used sparingly by most physicians because of their potential toxic effects. Other immunosuppressants are currently under study.

Special diets in vogue prior to the sulfasalazine era have given way to defined diets with glucose, fatty acids, and digests of protein. O'Morain in 1982 proposed an elemental diet as specific treatment of small-bowel Crohn's. Toxic megacolon and deaths from ulcerative colitis have become rare since good medical care and earlier surgery have been common practice. The cancer threat in long-term ulcerative colitis is less than originally thought, but still mandates meticulous surveillance for dysplasia, a harbinger of cancer. Meanwhile, in Crohn's disease, the old notion that wide resection of intestine can extirpate the disease has been replaced by minimalist surgery. Regrettably, cause, cure, or prevention of IBD remains as elusive as they were in Dalziel's time.

CHAPTER FIVE

Epidemiology of Inflammatory Bowel Disease

There is something fascinating about science. One gets such wholesome
returns of conjectures out of such trifling investment of fact.
                                                    Mark Twain (1835–1910)

"Epidemiology is that branch of Medical Science which treats of
epidemics" (Onions, 1973). It has come to mean the study of the
demography and geography of disease; that is, who has the disease
and where. It encompasses factors that might influence the occurrence of the disease, such as race, age, sex, and such environmental
factors as diet or pollution. This science has two principal purposes.
The first is to draw attention to the important diseases of mankind
so that resources may be mobilized to counter them. The current
public health emphasis on heart disease and cancer owes much to
epidemiologic evidence of their great prevalence and cost. Second,
epidemiologic study serves to point out associations with environmental factors that might increase our understanding of the disease,
and perhaps even help identify the cause and a means of prevention. The association of lung cancer to tobacco smoke is a classic
example.

   The epidemiology of inflammatory bowel disease (IBD) is
fascinating in itself. The great prevalence in western countries is all

the more poignant in that, unlike the diseases that predominate in the elderly, IBD is a chronic disease of youth. Regrettably, the curious demographic and geographic characteristics of IBD have not yet greatly enhanced our understanding of the cause or treatment of ulcerative colitis and Crohn's disease.

DEFINITIONS

Inflammatory bowel disease is said to be endemic in Europe and North America; that is, it is continuously present in the population. The prevalence of a disease is an estimate of how many people in a given population are affected. It is usually expressed as the number of cases per 100,000 people. For example, the prevalence of ulcerative colitis in Copenhagen, Denmark from 1962 to 1978 was estimated to be 117 cases per 100,000 people. The incidence of a disease is a record of the number of new cases occurring per year. In a chronic disease such as ulcerative colitis, the prevalence is much greater than the incidence. During the same period in Copenhagen, the incidence of colitis was 8.1 cases per 100,000 people per year. Incidence is never greater than prevalence, and the two are equal only when the disease or accident is rapidly fatal (for example, drowning).

SOURCE OF THE DATA

Some people are so sensitive they feel snubbed if an epidemic overlooks them.
Frank Hubbard (1868–1930)

In order that the incidence and prevalence figures be credible, meticulous record keeping is essential. One needs to know exactly the population at risk and the number of cases with the disease. Precise disease criteria must be employed to identify those in that population with the disease. Central record keeping is a characteristic of several European national health services, so their data are of better quality than those found in decentralized services such as those in North America. In Copenhagen, Denmark, the health records of the city's half million people are available and include all cases of IBD. Some studies, especially those from large American centers, rely on data from hospitals, so that the incidence and prevalence of IBD is underestimated. Also, since hospitalized patients are more ill, complications may be overestimated. This difficulty is demonstrated in the published data regarding the incidence of colon cancer complicating ulcerative colitis. In Copenhagen, this incidence is estimated to be 1.4 percent after 18 years, a figure similar to that of other studies in Europe. This contrasts with a cancer estimate of 10 percent after 10 years of disease reported from several North American and British centers, where only the severest or most complicated cases are seen and included in the population at risk.

EPIDEMIOLOGICAL FEATURES

In the last chapter we learned that ulcerative colitis and Crohn's disease are different from one another, and have very different pathologies. It is surprising, therefore, that the epidemiology of these two conditions is so similar. They both occur most frequently in people originating in Northern Europe, and are diseases of youth. They are similarly present in males and females, especially common in European and North American Jews, and unusual in blacks and Asians. The major difference between the two is that the incidence and prevalence of ulcerative colitis are static, whereas those of Crohn's disease seem to have increased. It is a further curiosity that once a person has been found to have one of these two diseases, immediate family members have a 10-fold increase in risk of either disease. The family member is more likely to have the same disease, but not necessarily so.

The incidence and prevalence of ulcerative colitis in Copenhagen were stated previously. In Oxford, England, they are 6.5 per 100,000 per year and 79.9 per 100,000, whereas in North Tees, England, they are 15.5 per 100,000 per year and 99 per 100,000, respectively. In contrast, a study from Baltimore, Maryland, reports an incidence of 2.5 per 100,000 per year, and no prevalence figures are available. The incidence of Crohn's disease is reported to be as many as 6 per 100,000 per year, whereas the prevalence ranges from 10 to 70 per 100,000. A fair estimate of the incidence and prevalence of IBD in Europe and probably North America is thus 15 to 20 cases per 100,000 per year and 150 to 200 per 100,000, respectively. In a city of 1 million people, one therefore might expect to find 1,500 to 2,000 cases, about equally divided between ulcerative colitis and Crohn's disease.

The figures are similar in men and women. It is said, though, that colitis is slightly more common in males, and Crohn's disease is slightly more common in females. Jews from northern Europe (Ashkenazi Jews) have as much as four times the risk of IBD compared with that of non-Jews, yet the incidence and prevalence of IBD in Israel, even among Jews from Europe, is less than that in North America and Europe. Blacks and Asians in the United States have less IBD than do their white compatriots, but those affected are said to have more severe disease. It most often commences between adolescence and 30 years but may occur at any age. Some studies suggest a second incidence peak in the sixth and seventh decades of life.

ENVIRONMENTAL FACTORS

There is an apparent geographic variation in the epidemiology of IBD in the United States. From hospital and mortality figures (the only data available), it has been noted that IBD is more common in the northern United States than in the South. The trends are the same for blacks and whites and for ulcerative colitis and Crohn's disease, suggesting that causative environmental factors may be the same for both diseases. The clustering of both these diseases in certain families supports this notion. The suggestion that these conditions are more common in urban populations and in higher socioeconomic groups may be incorrect, in that these groups have easier access to health care. The prevalence of colitis in rural Scotland is similar to that in British urban areas.

The relationship of IBD to cigarette smoking is curious. This habit is less prevalent in those with ulcerative colitis than in those without the disease, and an attack of colitis is often preceded by cessation of smoking. In contrast, smoking is positively related to Crohn's disease. Furthermore, smokers have more severe Crohn's than do nonsmokers. The significance of these data is unknown.

PROGNOSIS

The prognosis of IBD varies from individual to individual. The overall outlook is similar in Crohn's disease and ulcerative colitis, except that the latter may be cured by proctocolectomy. As a general rule, more-severe and extensive disease is likely to require more hospitalization, more surgery, and more time lost from work. Despite the statistics, the course of these diseases is unpredictable for the individual sufferer. Nevertheless, most can look forward to productive careers and satisfying social lives (see Chapter 18).

The 1985 Copenhagen study found survival in the first 10 years following a diagnosis of Crohn's disease to be similar to that of the normal population. In a given year, 45 percent of people with Crohn's disease were asymptomatic, 30 percent had low disease activity, and 25 percent had high disease activity. Surgery was performed in 33 percent of patients during the year of diagnosis and in 13 percent the year after. The operative rate was 3 percent per year thereafter. Work capacity was normal in 75 percent of patients, but despite treatment, a relapse can be expected within 10 years in 99 percent of cases. In one often-quoted 1981 study from Birmingham, England, mortality is reported to be increased twofold in Crohn's disease, compared with that in controls. Death resulted from the disease or its complications, of which digestive tract cancers and suicide were important.

In a Scottish study, the first attack of ulcerative colitis was mild in 68 percent, and involved only the distal colon in 78 percent (ulcerative proctitis or proctosigmoiditis). The overall mortality was 3 percent. Nevertheless, the long-term survival of patients with ulcerative colitis in these Scottish, largely rural patients was similar to that expected in the normal population. Exceptions were those who had a severe first attack or extensive ulcerative colitis, in whom the mortality was 23 percent. Sixty-eight percent of patient years were remission years.

Among the urban population of Copenhagen, survival is virtually unaffected by the presence of ulcerative colitis. Colectomy was done in 10 percent of individuals in the first year, 23 percent within 10 years, and 31 percent by 18 years. In a given year, 50 percent were asymptomatic, 30 percent had low activity, and 20 percent had high activity. The work capacity after 3 years was similar to that of controls, but the 10-year relapse rate among patients who did not have surgery was nearly 100 percent. Prognosis thus depends on many factors: the inclusion or not of all cases in the population studied, urban versus rural settings, and early versus late colectomy.

Unlike that for Crohn's disease, proctocolectomy for ulcerative colitis affords a complete cure, and, barring complications of the surgery, relapse no longer occurs. The cancer risk among those with ulcerative colitis in Copenhagen was only 1.4 percent over 18 years, a figure much lower than those usually quoted (see Chapter 17), because this study avoids the selection pitfalls found at most major centers. For example, ulcerative proctitis is included in most European studies of the epidemiology of ulcerative colitis, but largely excluded in tertiary referral centers, which deal with more serious and extensive disease. According to several studies, distal colitis or ulcerative proctitis is destined to extend further up the colon in only about 10 percent of adults, but the likelihood seems greater in children.

Without surgery, ulcerative colitis will almost certainly recur within 10 years, whereas in Crohn's disease, surgery may have little influence on recurrence. Nevertheless, at least one half of patients with ulcerative colitis and Crohn's disease remain asymptomatic within any given year. Furthermore, IBD appears to have less effect on work capacity and life expectancy than is generally believed. From placebo-controlled trials, it can be deduced that there is a natural tendency for the disease to remit, or stay in remission, in many instances. This natural history should encourage patience in treatment and discourage the overenthusiastic use of toxic drugs.

There is further discussion of prognosis and the quality of life in Chapter 18.

COST

No accurate estimate of the cost of IBD is available; however, the consumption of medical resources is considerable, because IBD tends to commence in youth and recur many times over a lifetime. In addition to the time lost from work, the investigation and treatment of this disease may be very expensive. Consultations, continuing medical care, imaging, and laboratory tests are required, not only initially, but also periodically through the course of the disease. Prolonged drug therapy is often necessary. Most sufferers will eventually require hospitalization and surgery, sometimes repeatedly. The care of 200 IBD patients per 100,000 people, is an important expense.

SUMMARY

The overall incidence of ulcerative colitis and Crohn's disease is 15 to 20 cases per 100,000 people per year, and the prevalence is 150 to 200 cases per 100,000 people. Ulcerative colitis is slightly more common, but the prevalence of Crohn's disease is increasing. Inflammatory bowel disease is similarly present in males and females. The two diseases are most prevalent in the inhabitants and the descendants of inhabitants of northern Europe, especially Jews. Uncommon now, IBD prevalence is increasing in Asians and blacks. The prognosis in terms of work capacity and recurrences is similar in ulcerative colitis and Crohn's disease, but only the former can be cured by colectomy. Even following surgery, the recurrence rate in Crohn's disease is nearly 100 percent over 10 years. With good medical care, it seems that life expectancy is little altered by either disease. Among all patients with ulcerative colitis, the incidence of colon cancer rises after 10 years.

CHAPTER SIX

Cause of Inflammatory Bowel Disease

To be consigned to a life spent searching for the aetiology of inflammatory bowel disease remains . . . a cause for supplication to St. Jude.

I. W. Booth, 1991

Discussion of the cause of inflammatory bowel disease (IBD) could be very short or very long. The short version is that we do not know the cause. A long answer would require an extensive knowledge of genetics, psychosomatic theory, microbiology, and immunology. I shall attempt to steer this discussion between these two extremes. Despite their epidemiologic similarities, and their similar responses to drugs, it is by no means certain that ulcerative colitis and Crohn's disease have the same cause. Nevertheless, discussions of etiology tend to lump the two together. A single cause for either seems improbable; it is more likely that many causative factors come together in a few susceptible individuals to produce disease. These putative factors, genetic, psychogenic, dietary, infectious, or immune, seem to be shared by both diseases.

CLINICAL OBSERVATIONS

Any explanation of the cause of IBD must take into account the observations of clinicians. The disease tends to be located where there is slowing or stasis of the flow of intestinal contents through the gut, such as above a sphincter. Ulcerative colitis invariably affects the area immediately above the anal sphincter. Crohn's disease usually is found above the ileocecal valve, in the perianal region, or in postoperative recurrences, just above where the bowel is rejoined (anastomosis). When the disease spreads, it tends to do so proximally, that is, toward the mouth.

In Crohn's disease, if a segment of bowel is bypassed surgically, and the fecal flow diverted, some healing occurs in the bypassed segment. Reconstitution of gut continuity results in rapid recurrence of the disease. In one study of patients with Crohn's colitis, the colon improved when protected from the fecal flow by an ileostomy. When the ileostomy effluent was then injected into the colon, there were soon signs of disease activity. This phenomenon could be prevented if the feces were finely filtered.

Elemental diets have been used in the treatment of Crohn's disease, with apparent success (Chapter 25). An elemental diet contains the basic sugar, amino acid, and fatty acid components of carbohydrate, protein, and fat. These nutrients are absorbed in the small intestine, and unlike whole foods, are not large enough to stimulate the immune system (nonantigenic), or provide a colon residue to feed the fecal bacteria. These observations foster the belief that there is something in the gut lumen (a luminal factor) that triggers the immune and inflammatory reactions seen in IBD. Such a factor in food or in the colon bacteria could act as an antigen to which the gut's immune system reacts inappropriately.

That the immune system is involved in IBD is supported by many other observations: the intense concentration in the angry, inflamed gut of cells that are known to participate in cellular or humeral immunity; the association of many extraintestinal manifestations of IBD that are believed to be due to disordered immunity (see Chapter 16); and the amelioration of the disease by drugs such as prednisone or 6-mercaptopurine (6-MP), which suppress the immune response.

Attacks of IBD are often blamed on upper respiratory infections or acute gastroenteritis, but usually no such trigger can be identified. It is curious that smoking is more common in those with Crohn's disease than in the nondiseased population. Indeed, smokers have more disease complications than do nonsmokers. Paradoxically, ulcerative colitis is more common in nonsmokers. There are also reports of increased Crohn's disease incidence in users of birth control pills. The importance of these observations in the causation of IBD is uncertain.

GENETICS

Data presented in the last chapter indicate genetic factors common to both types of IBD. Ulcerative colitis and Crohn's disease are most common in people native to northern Europe or their descendants, especially the Jews of northern Europe (Ashkenazi). Inflammatory bowel disease is much less common in blacks and Asians, although their IBD incidence seems to be increasing. There is increased likelihood of either ulcerative colitis or Crohn's disease in first-degree relatives of patients with IBD. Among monozygotic (identical) twins, the rate of concordance is even higher. In this case, the twin invariably has the same disease as the patient. In contrast, there is no evidence of increased risk of IBD among spouses of patients. This suggests that the increased risk in family members has a genetic rather than an environmental explanation.

In certain localities, tissue antigens such as those of the human leukocyte antigen (HLA) series seem to be common in IBD, but no specific worldwide antigen has been identified. There is certainly no obvious mendelian pattern of inheritance such as that seen with hemophilia or Tay–Sachs disease. It is yet possible that some people inherit a tendency to develop IBD, which becomes manifest when triggered by something in the environment: a stress, a microorganism, or an immune response to an intestinal antigen.

PSYCHOSOMATICS

The notion that ulcerative colitis is caused by a psychologic or psychiatric state was current in the 1930s, and echoes of this hypothesis are heard even now. It was based on observations of the sufferers' personalities. Engel described ulcerative colitis patients as obsessive–compulsive, immature, and dependent. Others have since pointed out that this disease often commences in adolescents, in whom urgent, painful, bloody stools and recurrent periods of illness might cause rather than result from the psychological distress. Enforced confinement for long periods in the toilet is bound to affect one's personality. Furthermore, many, perhaps most, patients with severe ulcerative colitis demonstrate no overt psychological disability. Mendeloff, in a survey of patients with ulcerative colitis, was unable to identify any psychological abnormality peculiar to those with the disease.

Alternatively, could a psychologic blow such as loss of one's job, marriage breakup, or death of a relative alter the balance of forces in the gut and trigger an attack? We know that depression, for example, may alter one's immune response. Mendeloff's work, and a recent study that found no psychologic precipitants of an IBD attack, cast doubt on this hypothesis. Nevertheless, our minds and bodies do not function independently, and whether cause or effect, psychologic distress is a very important component of IBD. It cannot be neglected in the treatment of either ulcerative colitis or Crohn's disease (see Chapter 18).

DIET

A belief exists, cherished by many sufferers, that IBD is due to something in the diet. Egged on by clinical ecologists, many exhaust much effort in the pursuit of the perfect diet. Sometimes, presumed offending foods are eliminated one by one until nutrition is threatened. Random attacks and spontaneous remissions that characterize the natural history of IBD reinforce the notion that some dietary transgression is at fault. At first glance, the apparent benefit of bowel rest, or an elemental diet that excludes nutrients large enough to trigger an immune response, seems to support the possibility of a dietary culprit. On the other hand, food withdrawal induces many other changes in the contents, flora, and immune activity of the bowel. Furthermore, on remission of the disease, the patient usually resumes his normal diet without untoward effect. Despite much research over many years, no plausible dietary factor has been identified.

Early reports of an intolerance to the milk sugar lactose during an acute attack of IBD have led many to omit milk from the diet. A principal source of calcium and vitamin D is thereby excluded. Such deprivation increases the risk of metabolic bone disease (osteoporosis and osteomalacia), especially in those who have small-bowel Crohn's or ileal resection. In most patients who do not have inherited lactose intolerance, withdrawal of milk is necessary only during an acute attack, if at all. Lactose has no causative role.

In one study of patients with Crohn's disease who achieved remission of their disease while on an elemental diet or parenteral (intravenous) nutrition, foods were reintroduced through a tube one at a time. Some reacted negatively to dairy products, wheat, meat, or other items. Most IBD specialists remain skeptical, however, and much more proof is required before patients should be subjected to the complicated testing and dietary advice this implies. Even this study does not claim that a single dietary factor causes all Crohn's disease. We humans are very suggestible, and a specific antifood bias may be difficult to overcome. We come to believe a food causes symptoms, and so it does. Nevertheless, proof that specific foods cause IBD is not forthcoming.

INFECTION

The bloody flux is a term from the prebacteriology era that was used to describe acute colitis. Typical features, we now know, may result from infection by numerous organisms including shigella and salmonella (see Chapter 9). Now these organisms are readily detected by routine bacteriologic testing of the stool. Several offending organisms were identified one by one late in the nineteenth century. Even recently, new causes of acute colitis have been found, namely campylobacter and enterohemorrhagic *Escherichia coli*. The remaining bloody fluxes for which no causative organism can be identified are said to be caused by ulcerative colitis. The possibility still exists that an organism, as yet unrecognized, might be the culprit. Even if colitis is an immune disorder, an organism might trigger the immune response in a susceptible individual.

In the 1800s, even well into the twentieth century, the inflamed, thickened terminal ileum and cecum so typical today of Crohn's disease would have been blamed on tuberculosis. With the virtual disappearance of that disease in western countries, intestinal tuberculosis is seldom encountered today. However, this history has nurtured the notion that a tuberculosislike organism (*Mycobacterium*) is at fault. This hypothesis is further reinforced by the presence of a similar organism in Crohn's-like lesions in goats. Nevertheless, the existing evidence does not favor an infectious cause for IBD.

If infection were responsible for IBD, several important observations would need to be reconciled. Although IBD tends to "cluster" in families, there is no evidence of transmission of the disease between spouses. Nurses and gastroenterologists are not at risk. Eradication of infection depends on the integrity of the gut's inflammatory and immune response. Why then should drugs that impair the immune response such as prednisone or 6-MP in fact improve the disease? Why are antibiotics ineffective in IBD? A causative organism must have unique characteristics to escape detection by modern laboratory techniques. Also, infection poorly explains the chronic, recurring nature of the disease.

Nevertheless, microorganisms cannot be ignored. Colon contents include myriad bacteria constituting the major proportion of fecal mass. Each organism has achieved an entente with the immune system, so it and the host may survive and thrive. In such a crowded environment, a single, chance bacteria/immune mismatch may trigger the chain of destructive gut events that we know as IBD.

IMMUNITY

Immunology is a fast-growing science. Altered immunity is an integral feature of many human diseases, including cancer, organ-transplant rejection, infection, rheumatic diseases, and skin eruptions. The subject can be given only cursory attention here. Many immune phenomena are found in patients with IBD, and altered immunity is believed to play a role in its pathogenesis. The nature of this role in relation to gut inflammation is not understood; therefore, one cannot yet determine whether the observed immune phenomena are causes, effects, or innocent bystanders.

There are two broad types of immunity: humeral and cellular. In the former, certain lymphocytes (white blood cells) produce proteins called gamma globulins, which are antibodies. Each antibody has its own specific antigen. These antibodies circulate in the blood and other body fluids and react on contact with foreign, or what they identify as foreign, proteins or antigens. The antigen–antibody reaction results in inactivation or destruction of the foreign substance by a variety of mechanisms as part of an inflammatory process. Examples of such foreign antigens in the gut are foods, bacterial components, and possibly even a person's own intestinal cells, somehow made antigenic. Cellular immunity refers to a process by which activated lymphocytes or *killer cells* ingest or destroy the foreign protein. The activities of these two types of immune response are carefully regulated and are vital to the body's integrity. Nowhere is this more critical than in the gut.

The gut is well equipped to mount an immune response. The area under the epithelium is densely populated with mononuclear cells, notably lymphocytes, which are capable of responding to any foreign threat. Like a customs post, the gut mucosa must admit material that is nutrient, while rejecting and possibly destroying invasive material that might do harm. While harmful bacteria (pathogens) are resisted, the billions of normally harmless bacteria that populate our gut are tolerated, so long as they remain within the lumen. The mix of tolerated bacteria is determined early in life, and every individual achieves a personal detente with a bacterial flora unique to his or her colon. There are many opportunities for the immune system to misfire, and produce a destructive inflammation. Nevertheless, some still claim that IBD represents a normal immune response to some gut pathogen, such as a microorganism or a ingested protein that has hitherto escaped detection.

Another concept is that of autoimmunity. The immune system is apparently capable of attacking *self*, that is, the individual's own intestinal epithelial cells. Such self-destruction might occur if antigens in the gut lumen so closely resemble epithelial cell antigens that the immune system mistakenly attacks them. Alternatively, mucosal or epithelial antigens may become altered in some way, so that they become "foreign" and an immunologic target. Cited as evidence for an autoimmune process in IBD is the presence of anticolon antibodies in the blood sera of patients with ulcerative colitis, and the association of IBD with other diseases of presumed autoimmunity.

A recent hypothesis is that IBD is a disorder of immunoregulation. In normal animals, the mucosa is said to undergo a constant, low-grade, controlled inflammation, the result of ongoing local immune skirmishes. This activity may be in response to the luminal presence of foreign bacterial or dietary antigens that threaten the individual's integrity. Of interest, local gut inflammation is less in animals nurtured in a germ-free environment. According to this hypothesis, the normal immune-suppressor activity fails in IBD, and an uncontrolled immune reaction generates excessive inflammation that destroys normal gut tissue.

Whatever mechanism proves to be correct, the result of the immunologic process is a destructive acute and chronic inflammation of the gut. This implies activation of the white blood cells (lymphocytes and polymorphs) in the mucosa and the release of chemical mediators of inflammation and cell damage. The latter include the products of arachadonic acid metabolism, prostaglandins, and leukotrienes, which are in turn inhibited by drugs commonly used to treat IBD, such as prednisone and 5-aminosalicylic acid (5-ASA). Moreover, the immune system itself may be suppressed by prednisone and the immunosuppressive drugs (see Chapters 20 to 22).

SUMMARY

The cause of IBD is unknown. Ulcerative colitis and Crohn's disease may have different causes despite their similarities in epidemiology, genetics, and therapy. In either case, there are undoubtedly several causative factors. Any explanation must embrace evidence that a luminal factor seems important, that either disease is likely in families of patients with IBD, that spouses and medical personnel are not at increased risk, and that antiinflammatory and immunosuppressive drugs appear to be beneficial. There does appear to be a genetic predisposition to the disease. Psychologic and sociologic factors influence how the patient copes with IBD, but probably play little role in its cause. No organism has been identified consistently in IBD patients, and there is little support for a contagion. The smart money is now invested in the immune system, whose inappropriate activity, triggered by unknown factors (perhaps in the gut lumen), sets off the severe acute and chronic gut inflammations that we recognize as ulcerative colitis and Crohn's disease.

PART TWO
Ulcerative Colitis

CHAPTER SEVEN

Ulcerative Colitis
Pathology and Pathogenesis

Pathology would remain a lovely science even if there were no therapeutics, just as seismology is a lovely science, though no one knows how to stop earthquakes.

H. L. Mencken (1880–1956)

Ulcerative colitis is an acute and chronic inflammation of the colon extending a variable distance from the anus, and characterized by recurrent attacks interspersed among periods of low or no activity. The cause is unknown, but the anatomical changes in the colon (pathology) are well recognized, and help explain the genesis of symptoms. At least until the very late stages of the disease, the inflammation is confined to the inner, mucosal layer of the colon. There are several variants of the disease, depending on the extent of colon involvement: *proctitis*; *proctosigmoiditis*; *left-sided colitis*; and *pancolitis* (Chapter 3). This chapter discusses the pathology of ulcerative colitis, and how this pathology causes symptoms.

OTHER COLON INFLAMMATIONS

As we shall see shortly, inflammation is a response of the tissues to injury. Thus many agents that attack the colon may elicit an inflammatory response. Examples include bacterial infections such as salmonella, shigella or campylobacter; parasites such as ameba; a ruptured colon diverticulum resulting in abscess (diverticulitis); and radiation. Some organisms such as shigella produce mucosal changes that are very similar to those of ulcerative colitis; thus, when the disease first strikes, diagnosis must await the results of stool cultures. Unlike ulcerative colitis, enteric infections rarely recur or become chronic. Inflammation due to radiation injury or diverticulitis is usually distinct from that of ulcerative colitis.

Crohn's disease may affect the colon, but differs from ulcerative colitis in many respects. Sparing of the rectum, perianal disease, granuloma, and fistula are more common in the former, and only in Crohn's may the small bowel be affected. Also in Crohn's, all three layers of the gut are involved, and complicating carcinoma seems to be less likely. In the early stages of the disease, especially if it is very severe, we may not be able to determine whether ulcerative colitis or Crohn's disease is present. This *indeterminate* colitis usually declares itself in time, but occasionally the final diagnosis is made at surgery. Further discussion is found later in this book.

PATHOLOGY

Ugliness is a point of view: an ulcer is wonderful to a pathologist.
A. O'Malley (1858–1932)

During an acute attack of ulcerative colitis, the colon mucosa shows the features of acute inflammation. Through a sigmoidoscope or colonoscope, the examiner may see a diffuse redness that obscures the normal blood vessel pattern of the colon inner surface. Tiny pits may be seen, which represent the ulcers, and in more severe cases, there will be blood and pus exuding through the ulcers. Later the ulcers may become confluent, and eroded mucosa may leave islands of relatively normal mucosa called *pseudopolyps*.

Under microscopic examination of a biopsy, one might first see an infiltration of acute multinucleated inflammatory cells called polymorphonuclear leukocytes, a type of white blood cell that accumulates from the bloodstream in response to tissue injury. These *polymorphs* are the major component of pus. Blood flow to the mucosa increases, and damage to the blood vessels leads to hemorrhage and congestion of the tissues with red blood cells. This accounts for the redness, swelling, and bleeding seen by the endoscopist. The inflammatory cells crowd around the crypts, and a crypt full of white blood cells is known as a *crypt abscess* (Figure 7-1). Although typical of ulcerative colitis, crypt abscesses are found in infections as well. Other cells involved in the inflammatory process secrete chemicals that may participate in the destruction of colon epithelium. The resultant destruction produces ulcers or defects in the colon epithelium through which blood and protein leak into the lumen.

In more severe cases, the ulcers deepen, widen, and coalesce, leaving islands of intact but inflamed epithelium (Figure 7-2). As described, these pseudopolyps appear as small tumors or polyps to the endoscopist. Although the muscle layers of the colon are not directly involved in the inflammatory process, they tend to contract, producing a thickened, shortened colon. The normal haustra are flattened, giving the colon the appearance on x-ray of a rigid, featureless tube (Figures 8-2 and 10-5, pages 85 and 110). The normal braking action of the colon is lost. Sometimes narrowing (stricture) of the colon occurs, causing the physician to worry about a complicating cancer (Figure 10-4, page 109).

The colon mucosa has great powers of repair. After an acute attack, the mucosa may reconstitute itself completely. When such a remission occurs, the examining endoscopist may be unable to detect any sign of disease, and even the pathologist may find little evidence of colitis in a biopsy. In severe, chronic disease, however, some changes become permanent. The ulcers may heal, but rigidity of the colon, loss of vascular pattern, and pseudopolyps remain as footprints of colitis past and harbingers of colitis yet to come.

One reason for the great restorative powers of the colon is the rapidity with which the epithelium regenerates itself. Rapid epithe-

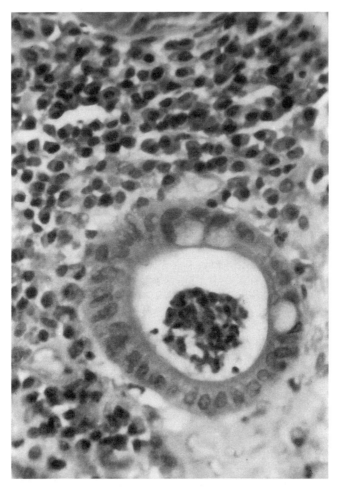

Figure 7-1. Crypt abscess. This is a photomicrograph of the colon submucosa of a patient with acute colitis. The tissues are crowded with inflammatory cells. The circular ring of cells is a crypt in which some pus cells have collected.

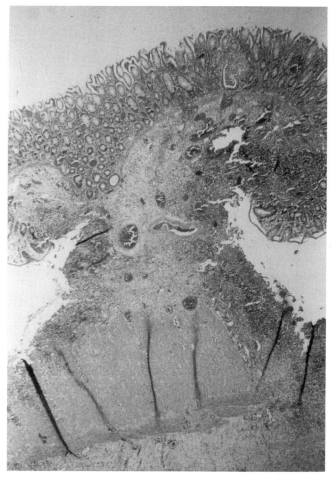

Figure 7-2. Pseudopolyp. This is an island of inflamed but intact mucosa in a sea of ulceration. It is, therefore, not a true polyp.

lial cell regeneration and the surrounding inflammation increase the opportunity for fundamental cell change. This is doubtless the reason that colon cancer is a greater-than-normal risk in ulcerative colitis. A change in the appearance of the epithelial cells, called *dysplasia*, is an important early sign of a complicating colon cancer (see Chapter 17). In dysplasia the epithelial cells appear abnormal, with large, disorderly nuclei signifying increased cell reproduction (mitosis) and darkened cell fluid (cytoplasm). A pathologist skilled in gastrointestinal disease is required to distinguish dysplasia from the effects of inflammation, but when dysplasia is present, there must be a strong suspicion of imminent or actual colon cancer. After the disease has been present 10 years, the risk of malignant change in the colon mucosa is greater than that in those without colitis; thus, many experts recommend regular colonoscopies with biopsies. Colectomy is done if persistent dysplasia is found. Others caution that the finding of dysplasia may be too late a phenomenon on the road to cancer. They recommend colectomy in long-standing, continuously active colitis in order to remove the chance of cancer.

PATHOGENESIS

The term *pathogenesis* is usually used to denote the means by which disease manifests itself. Although the cause of ulcerative colitis is unknown (see Chapter 6), the pathology we have just described can explain how the symptoms are generated. The bleeding results from the increased colon mucosal blood flow, damaged blood vessels, and release of red blood cells through the ulcerated epithelium. The colon normally salvages about 1 liter of the fluid daily presented to it by the small bowel. In ulcerative colitis the damaged mucosa is unable to absorb this fluid, and watery diarrhea may occur. The inflamed, ulcerated mucosa leaks protein-rich serum and pus. Impaired colon motility, characterized by increased peristaltic contractions, is experienced by the patient as cramps, and a lack of segmenting or braking action in the sigmoid further aggravates the diarrhea. The result in acute disease is a bloody, watery, pusy, crampy diarrhea. In the chronic state, there may be less loss of blood and pus, but the mucosa may still be damaged. The rigid, nonabsorbing colon becomes a mere tube or sluice for the exit of small-bowel fluid.

The inflamed rectal mucosa and the increased intestinal fluid with which it must cope create a sense of urgency to defecate. If urgency is accompanied by spasm of the rectal muscles, the result is a painful urge to defecate called *tenesmus*. This is a sign of severe colitis.

The toxicity associated with inflammation of large areas of the colon has general effects. Chemical transmitters exuded by inflammatory cells cause fever, malaise, and suppression of red blood cell production in the bone marrow. With the superimposed blood loss, and perhaps red cell destruction (hemolysis) resulting from drugs, an anemia may result, with its accompanying weakness, breathlessness, and even chest pain. Poor appetite or fear of eating, plus the loss of protein from the gut, result in weight loss and low blood protein (albumin). In severe cases, the colon muscle becomes paralyzed, dilates (*toxic megacolon*), and if urgent action is not taken, the colon may perforate. If the fluid loss is great, dehydration may result.

SUMMARY

The inflammation of ulcerative colitis is confined to the mucosa of the colon. Thus, removal of the colon cures the disease. Unlike Crohn's disease, the muscular and serosal layers are not involved. This inflammation accounts for the symptoms. Failure of the colon mucosa to absorb water presented to it from the ileum, loss of blood, pus, and albumin through the ulcers, and abnormal performance of colon muscle layers account for the profuse, bloody, pusy, crampy diarrhea so typical of this disease. The inflammation, if active and extending beyond the rectum, may cause systemic symptoms such as fever, anemia, weight loss, and malaise. When the disease is extensive and severe, and extends into the deeper layers of the colon, complications such as toxic megacolon, massive hemorrhage, and perforation are likely to occur.

CHAPTER EIGHT

Ulcerative Colitis

Symptoms and Diagnosis

> As no two persons are exactly alike in health so neither are any two in
> disease; and no diagnosis is complete or exact which does not include
> an estimate of the personal character or the constitution of the patient.
>
> Sir James Paget (1814–1899)

The cardinal symptom of ulcerative colitis is diarrhea, usually with
blood and pus, but the disease is very variable from individual to
individual, both in its manifestations and in its course. Symptoms
are directly related to the extent and intensity of the colon inflammation. Pancolitis thus is likely to produce more severe symptoms than
proctitis, and a severe inflammation with coalesced ulcers, pseudopolyps, and strictures results in more intense local and systemic
symptoms than does mild or inactive disease. It is important to keep
these relationships in mind as we consider symptoms, but there are
two other important considerations. Patients are all individuals and
as such react individually to disease. It is common for the perceptive
physician to observe that some individuals with severe disease
pursue their lives with prodigious fortitude, even to the point of
denial, while others are incapacitated by a seemingly negligible
proctitis (see Chapter 18). Finally, 15 to 20 percent of otherwise

healthy individuals have the periodic abdominal pain and altered bowel habit of an irritable bowel syndrome. Doubtless this occurs in ulcerative colitis as well, and may delay recognition of the disease on the one hand, or pose as an attack of colitis on the other. With these factors in mind, let us consider the clinical manifestations and diagnosis of the disease.

SYMPTOMS OF ULCERATIVE COLITIS

Bowel Symptoms

An attack of ulcerative colitis usually begins with diarrhea. It may commence slowly with loose bowel movements, or with startling rapidity, mimicking an attack of infectious colitis. The more extensive the disease, the more impaired the salt and water absorption in the colon, and the greater the diarrhea. The appearance of blood and pus in the stool signals the development of ulcers and is a measure of the intensity of the inflammation. Although not directly affected by the inflammatory activity in the mucosa, the muscle layer of the colon functions abnormally, resulting in impaired braking action and vigorous peristalsis, to rid the gut of irritants. The vigorous peristaltic colon contractions are perceived as cramps and may be very intense. Fluid feces trickling into the sensitive, inflamed rectum exaggerates the stimulus to defecation, and a powerful urge may become the dominant symptom. When the urge to defecate becomes painful because of rectal and anal spasm, it is known as *tenesmus* and is considered a sign of severe disease.

There are variations of this attack. In proctitis, only the distal few centimeters of the bowel are affected, and constipation may dominate, as if the colon is reluctant to permit stool to enter the affected area. When hard, constipated stools do pass an inflamed rectum, they are coated with blood and pus. Conversely, in extensive disease, with mild inflammation, there may be diarrhea, but little or no blood. Unlike those in Crohn's disease, anal lesions such as fissures, fistulas, and abscesses are uncommon, but the increased stool traffic may excoriate the skin around the anus. This results in itching, and often painful passage of stool.

The pain may become steady and severe, rather than crampy, with abdominal tenderness, fever, and malaise. This indicates severe disease with either an inflated colon, or inflammation of the outer coat of the gut (serosa) and impending perforation. These may be signs of fulminant colitis or toxic megacolon (Chapter 10). The diarrhea may seem to improve, but in this setting, less bowel action may be an ominous sign. In contrast, with complete remission of the disease, cramps and altered bowel habits may occur because of a coexistent irritable bowel. Such symptoms must not be mistaken for, or treated as, colitis.

Systemic Symptoms

Inflammation, however local, may result in symptoms affecting the entire body. Even an infected thumb initiates an inflammatory response that may cause systemic symptoms. The inflamed tissue, and the cells that participate in the inflammation, release toxins and chemical mediators into the bloodstream with profound systemic effects. The commonest are fever, malaise, feeling of weakness, and fatigue. Blood loss and toxic depression of the bone marrow produce anemia, which adds to the malaise. Cramps and diarrhea disrupt the sleep pattern. Appetite is suppressed, and energy is consumed by the inflammation. Eating is feared, because it stimulates the already oversensitive gut. Weight loss is therefore common. All these may occur in mild to moderate ulcerative colitis.

In very severe disease, the systemic manifestations become even more profound. Fluid and salt loss from the colon lead to dehydration and decreased blood levels of sodium and potassium. Fever and malaise may progress to prostration and shock. If the disease becomes fulminant, delirium may intervene. Nutrition becomes impaired, and the body's ability to cope with the demands of the inflammation are compromised. Protein loss in the gut and poor diet cause the blood protein (albumin) to decrease. If urgent measures are not employed, death may ensue. Such progression of colitis to the brink of death is avoidable with appropriate medical treatment and timely colectomy, and should never occur with contemporary care.

Every disease inspires a psychological response. The reaction may be rage, anxiety, fear, depression, stubborn denial, or passive resentment. In the absence of faith, someone or something must shoulder the blame, whether it be self, family, caregiver, or the environment. Coping with such normal human reactions can profoundly affect the systemic effects of any disease, and ulcerative colitis is no exception. Against a background of such emotion, the optimal treatment of colitis requires a skillful doctor and an insightful patient (Chapter 18).

Extraintestinal Manifestations

The many extraintestinal manifestations of inflammatory bowel disease (IBD) are discussed in Chapter 16. The reader should be aware that associated diseases, such as sclerosing cholangitis or rheumatoid spondylitis, may add to the systemic effects of ulcerative colitis. Unwanted effects of drugs, such as steroids, sulfasalazine, or nonsteroidal analgesics used in IBD or its extraintestinal manifestations, may further aggravate the patient's general condition.

SIGNS OF ULCERATIVE COLITIS

What the examining physician observes to be abnormal in a patient is called a physical sign. In mild ulcerative colitis there may be no sign at all. Sometimes there is tenderness over the colon, especially above the left groin where the sigmoid colon is near the surface. Excoriations around the anus and blood and pus on the examination of the rectum with the finger suggest ulcerative colitis, in the context of a suggestive history of bloody diarrhea and cramps.

In moderate to severe disease there may be pallor of the skin and tongue (anemia), elevated temperature, and signs of recent weight loss. Some extraintestinal manifestations, such as eye inflammation (iritis) or red nodules on the shins (erythema nodosum), may herald an attack. The patient may appear depressed or anxious. When the disease becomes fulminant, the abdomen is distended and very tender to touch. Bowel sounds heard through the stethoscope are hyperactive. With toxic megacolon or perforation of the colon, the distended large bowel becomes silent, the abdomen rigid, and signs of shock intervene, such as low blood pressure, weak rapid pulse, flaccid muscles, extreme pallor, blue extremities, and altered consciousness. At this point, colectomy is overdue.

PROGNOSIS

The course of the disease is very variable. An initial attack may resolve without trace, only to return months, years, or even decades later. Successive attacks suffered by one individual may be carbon copies of one another, or they may be very different. In the case of a single attack, one may remain uncertain whether it was IBD rather than an infectious disease, even if the stool cultures are negative. Here one must await a recurrence, which is likely, indeed almost inevitable, in IBD. Often the remission is not complete, and minimal symptoms persist, accompanied by continued, low-grade colon inflammation. Occasionally remission does not occur. The disease may worsen despite expert treatment and require urgent surgery. In others, the colitis may simply continue so that treatment cannot be withdrawn, and elective surgery is required. Ulcerative colitis present for 10 years or more carries with it an increased risk of colon cancer. This and other factors affecting prognosis are discussed under complications (Chapter 10).

Ulcerative proctitis is a special case. Blood and pus in the stool may be alarming, and stubborn to treat. However, there are no systemic symptoms in proctitis, and the risk of cancer is probably no greater than that in unaffected people. It may persist for many years. Proctitis is destined to spread proximally up the colon in about 10 percent of cases after 5 to 10 years. In these cases the result is genuine ulcerative colitis with all its symptoms and risks.

DIAGNOSIS

In an initial attack of bloody diarrhea, the physician suspects the disease when he or she sees an inflamed rectum through a sigmoidoscope (see Figures 27-3, 27-4, and 27-5). With this instrument he or she is in a position to evaluate the extent and severity of the disease. The rectum is almost invariably involved in ulcerative colitis and, with a sigmoidoscope or colonoscope, one can determine the upper margin of the disease and classify it as proctitis, proctosigmoiditis, left-sided colitis, or pancolitis. At a minimum the normal blood vessel pattern of the colon inner surface (mucosa) is obscured by a diffuse redness. The bright, glistening mucosa becomes replaced by a dull, granular surface produced by a dense profusion of minute ulcers. Tiny bleeding points are seen in some deeper ulcers. In more severe disease, the ulcers are more obvious, and blood and pus occupy the lumen. In very severe disease, the normally contracting, valved, and convoluted colon becomes rigid, tubelike, and foreshortened. The ulcers coalesce, and tiny lumps of surviving mucosa appear as pseudopolyps.

In a young person, the principal conditions that may resemble ulcerative colitis are irritable bowel, Crohn's colitis, and infectious colitis. In the former, the rectosigmoid is normal on sigmoidoscopic examination, and there are no systemic signs. In Crohn's, the rectum may be spared, the involvement may be patchy, and there may be disease in the small bowel. Initial management is similar for ulcerative colitis and Crohn's colitis, so early differentiation is not essential. A more detailed account of Crohn's disease is found in Part 3. For practical purposes in the young, the main source of confusion with ulcerative colitis is infectious colitis.

In any acute attack of colitis, especially the first, the physician must exclude an infectious cause. The principal therapeutic drug for moderate to severe colitis is one of the adrenocorticoid steroids, such as prednisone. This impairs immunity and resistance to infection, and should be avoided with enteric (bowel) infections. A great many

TABLE 8-1
Some Infectious Causes of Colitis

Left colon	Campylobacter
	Salmonella
	Shigella
	Clostridium difficile
	Enterohemorrhagic *Escherichia coli*
	Gonococcus
	Entamoeba histolytica (a protozoan)
Right colon	Yersinia
	Campylobacter

organisms may cause a colitis. The common ones are listed in Table 8-1. Some deserve special mention. Amoebic dysentery is uncommon in urban North America or Europe, but is common in the Third World. The sigmoidoscopic appearance of amoebic colitis is distinct from that of ulcerative colitis. The ulcers are large, and undermine the adjacent mucosa. Normal-appearing mucosa lies between the ulcers. A bacteriologist, directly examining the stool, will usually discover the offending amoeba (*Entamoeba histolytica*).

Most colonic pathogens produce a colitis similar to ulcerative colitis. Some pathologists claim there are histologic features in the mucosa, such as more polymorphs and less crypt disruption, that distinguish infectious from noninfectious colitis. Few clinicians would depend on this, however. Thus the doctor must rely on the lack of a history suggestive of infection, a careful bacteriological analysis, and observation of the behavior of the process over several weeks or months in order to make a firm diagnosis of ulcerative colitis.

Some features in a patient's history might offer clues to certain infections. Shigella, the classic bacillary dysentery, often occurs as an epidemic in institutions, especially those for the mentally retarded, where personal hygiene is poor. Salmonella infections are acquired from undercooked poultry and eggs, or from a restaurant where the cook is a carrier. One type of *Escherichia coli* may be acquired from undercooked ground beef and cause a severe colitis. When one travels to tropical climes, he or she may acquire one of several enteric infections, an unwanted souvenir. The usual traveler's diarrhea is due to a small-bowel toxin produced by toxigenic *E. coli.* In this case the colon is unaffected, and the diarrhea is not bloody; however, salmonella, campylobacter, shigella, and *Entamoeba histolytica* may inflict on the traveler a colitis that mimics ulcerative colitis.

> Travel broadens the mind and opens the bowels.
> Sherwood Gorbach

In most of North America, *Campylobacter jejuni* is the commonest cause of bacterial colitis. This organism is often acquired from infected pets or farm animals. A man's dog may not, in this case, be his best friend. Sometimes campylobacter colitis is confined to the ileocecal region, and sigmoidoscopic examination will not discover it. Most commonly in Europe, Yersinia infection also affects the ileocecal region, and is occasionally mistaken for acute Crohn's ileocolitis.

Antibiotic therapy for an unrelated infection may permit overgrowth of *Clostridium difficile,* a toxin-producing organism that causes a characteristic *pseudomembranous colitis.* Common offenders are clindamycin, ampicillin, and amoxicillin. The sigmoidoscope reveals a patchy grey-yellow pseudomembrane, and mucosal biopsy is diagnostic. The diagnosis is confirmed by assay of the *C. difficile* toxin from the stool. This toxigenic colitis sometimes follows the cessation of the antibiotic by more than a month, and is also acquired, from other patients in hospital. Curiously this antibiotic-induced colitis is treated with another antibiotic, either metronidazole or vancomycin. Recurrences occur in 25 percent of cases, increasing its likelihood of confusion with IBD.

Homosexual men, with and without acquired immunodeficiency syndrome (AIDS), are susceptible to many enteric infections. Reinfection is common, so that if the sexual proclivities of the patient are unknown, a mistaken diagnosis of IBD may be established. Any of the previously mentioned organisms may be responsible for bowel disease in homosexuals, along with several others, such as gonorrhea.

Although negative stool cultures are crucial for the initial diagnosis of ulcerative colitis, there are pitfalls. Unless the specimens are collected early, the organisms may not be detected. Sometimes a relapse of ulcerative colitis may be precipitated by an enteric infection. Some laboratories do not routinely search for less common pathogens. Some organisms, such as that causing gonorrhea, are notoriously difficult to detect; thus, a thorough history, observation, good clinical judgment, and careful bacteriology are keys to diagnosis.

When colitis has its onset in the elderly, there are other considerations in the differential diagnosis. In those with severe cardiovascular disease, one might suspect ischemic colitis. In this disease, the colon is inflamed and congested because of poor blood circulation. Usually an ischemic gut causes much pain with rectal bleeding, and mucosal edema is recognized by endoscopy, x-ray, and biopsy. The rectum is seldom involved, and the disease may occur near the splenic flexure, where the margins of the blood supplies from the inferior and superior mesenteric arteries meet. Diverticulitis, infection due to a burst diverticulum in the sigmoid colon, causes pain and fever, but not usually bloody diarrhea. Rectal bleeding from colon carcinoma, adenomatous polyp, uninfected diverticulum, or other source occurs without fever, pus, or pain. A large villous adenoma of the rectum may produce blood and puslike mucus. Removal of this usually benign tumor is curative.

INVESTIGATION

A complete discussion of the investigational procedures an ulcerative colitis patient may undergo appears in Chapter 27. In the irritable bowel, blood tests such as the white blood cell count, platelet count, and erythrocyte sedimentation rate are normal, whereas they are usually abnormal in IBD. The serum albumin may be depressed. Stool examination for pathogens has already been discussed.

A plain x-ray of the abdomen may show gas shadows typical of ulcerative colitis (Figure 8-1), or characteristic features of other conditions such as Crohn's or ischemic colitis. It is very useful in the identification of megacolon or perforation (Chapter 10). A barium enema, in which barium is injected through the anus into the colon

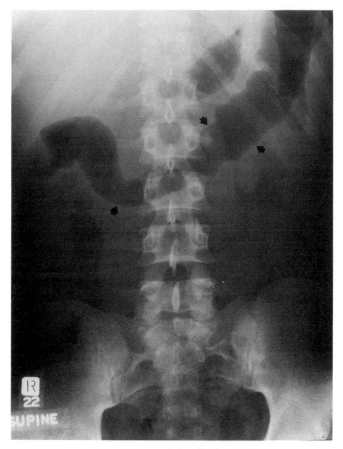

Figure 8-1. Plain x-ray of the abdomen in a patient presenting with acute colitis. The transverse colon is full of gas and shows on the film as a dark shadow indicated by arrows. Compare this with the transverse colon shown on the barium enema in Figure 27-9 and note that the normal segmental or haustral pattern is lost. In some places the colon appears as a rigid, featureless tube.

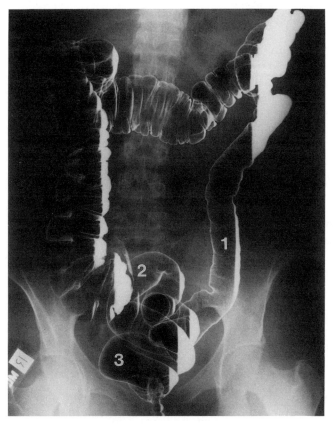

Figure 8-2. Barium enema in a patient with left-sided ulcerative colitis. Tiny ulcers can be seen along the descending colon (1), sigmoid colon (2), and rectum (3). The descending colon has lost its haustra. Each white spot within the affected colon represents barium pooling in a tiny mucosal ulcer. The ascending and transverse colon are nomal. Compare these features to the normal colon as seen in Figure 27-9.

while x-ray pictures are taken, provides a permanent record of the colon abnormalities (Figure 8-2), although subtle mucosal changes are sometimes missed. An x-ray of the small bowel contrasted by barium delivered from above should be normal in ulcerative colitis (Figure 27-8). Occasionally in pancolitis, a short segment of the terminal ileum may be distended and featureless, a reversible phenomenon known as *backwash ileitis*.

The most useful tool for the initial recognition of ulcerative colitis, and the monitoring of its progress, is sigmoidoscopy. With a rigid sigmoidoscope, one may examine only 15 to 25 centimeters of colon, and this instrument is seldom used now by gastroenterologists. Nevertheless, because the rectum is almost always representative of the disease, this venerable instrument is serviceable when a fiberoptic instrument is unavailable. The fiberoptic sigmoidoscope is 60 centimeters in length, and permits examination of the left colon, often as far as the splenic flexure. Colonoscopes are 160 centimeters or more in length, and allow whole-colon evaluation. Colonoscopy is a useful technique to determine the extent of the colitis, distinguish it from Crohn's, and obtain periodic screening biopsies for cancer.

SUMMARY

The cardinal feature of ulcerative colitis is bloody diarrhea. The patient is ill in proportion to the extent and severity of the disease; thus, ulcerative proctitis is unassociated with systemic symptoms, but severe pancolitis is associated with fever, anemia, malaise, and increased likelihood of complications. The most important diagnostic test after a good history is sigmoidoscopic observation of the typical changes in the rectum. In an acute attack in a young person, the disease must be distinguished from the irritable bowel, Crohn's colitis, and most important, enteric infections. In older patients, ischemic colitis, diverticulitis, and colon neoplasms may need consideration. The diagnosis should not be made without sigmoidoscopy. Colonoscopy, or occasionally barium enema, is eventually necessary to determine the extent of the disease and to screen for cancer.

CHAPTER NINE

Ulcerative Colitis

Treatment

Ulcerative colitis usually manifests itself in attacks, recurring perhaps one or twice a year, with relatively quiescent periods in between. A treatment strategy should include appropriate but vigorous treatment of attacks, and either maintenance or prophylaxis with a minimum of drugs through the quiet periods. This generally implies treatment with large doses of 5-aminosalicylic acid (5-ASA) compounds or corticosteroids when there is acute fever, cramps, and bloody diarrhea, and their replacement with smaller prophylactic doses of 5-ASA during remission. Along with supportive methods, these two drugs have been validated in the treatment of ulcerative colitis. Several other drugs have been shown to be effective in certain types of Crohn's disease, but this is not the case in ulcerative colitis. This chapter outlines the special therapeutic dilemmas that occur during the first attack of colitis, and describes a treatment response graded according to the severity of the attack and the extent of the disease. The treatment of complications is considered in the next chapter. The rationale of prophylaxis is also discussed, recognizing that attacks, remissions, and complications are phases in a disease continuum. While there is general agreement on the principles of therapy, physicians may vary in the details.

The drugs, diets, and operations employed in the treatment of ulcerative colitis are explained briefly in this chapter. A more detailed exposition of their rationale and undesirable effects appears in the last section of this book. It is an important fact that prednisone, the most effective drug in inflammatory bowel disease (IBD), has many undesirable effects, especially over time. One should therefore continually seek the lowest dose of prednisone that controls disease activity, and not miss the opportunity to discontinue the drug when remission has been achieved.

THE FIRST ATTACK

In a first attack of crampy, bloody diarrhea, the physician's first dilemma is to make the correct diagnosis. Prednisone, the mainstay of treatment of moderate and severe ulcerative colitis, suppresses the body's defenses to infection, so its use is clearly a mistake in the various infectious colitides described in the previous chapter. Sigmoidoscopy may permit one to diagnose colitis, but not usually to identify its cause. How, then, can the patient be managed while one awaits the results of stool cultures?

This is not usually difficult. Most colon infections are not treated with antibiotics unless the attack is very severe, or the organism is detected in the bloodstream. Supportive measures, such as rest, reduced food intake, rehydration through oral or intravenous fluid and salt solutions, and careful use of antidiarrhea drugs, are the same whether the colitis is infectious or not. The 5-ASA compounds do not adversely affect infection, so full doses may be started with impunity, and stopped if the diagnosis is not ulcerative colitis. When the negative stool culture results are available, usually 2 to 3 days later, a more confident diagnosis of ulcerative colitis is possible, and one may add or switch to prednisone if necessary.

In a recurrent attack, one is less likely to doubt the diagnosis of ulcerative colitis. On occasion, however, a bona fide attack may be precipitated by an enteric infection; therefore, if any suspicion of infection exists from a careful history, a stool culture is warranted.

The possibility that the first attack of colitis is due to Crohn's disease poses less dilemma, at least initially. At this stage, the two types of IBD are treated in a similar manner. Only later, when surgery or drugs more specific for Crohn's disease, such as 6-mercaptopurine (6-MP) are contemplated, does the distinction matter.

ULCERATIVE PROCTITIS

Proctitis involves only the rectum, and the upper margin of the disease is usually less than 20 centimeters from the anus (see Figure 3-1). The patient characteristically passes blood and mucus, often separate from or coating the stool. Diarrhea is usually not prominent. Paradoxically, there may even be constipation. Systemic signs such as fever and weight loss are usually absent. The endoscopist observes inflammation in the rectum indistinguishable from ulcerative colitis, except that it stops abruptly about 10 to 15 centimeters into the rectum. In 10 percent of patients with ulcerative proctitis, the disease eventually extends beyond the rectum, so one should be alert to bloody diarrhea, weight loss, and fever.

Proctitis is not a serious condition. It does not disable, or lead to the complications of ulcerative colitis; accordingly, the treatment should not do more harm than the disease. Patients are seldom ill, so supportive needs are minimal. Hospitalization, diet restriction, or intravenous treatment are not necessary. Systemic steroids or immunoregulatory drugs that might be used for more extensive colitis are overkill and inappropriate here. Because the rectum is easily accessible to enemas and suppositories, local treatment makes sense. Suppositories of 5-ASA are available in 250-milligram and 500-milligram strength (Salofalk). If administered two or three times a day, they may control the disease. If this fails, a steroid suppository may help [hydrocortisone acetate (Cortament 10 or 40 milligrams)]. There are 4-gram 5-ASA enemas (Salofalk) and steroid enemas (eg, betamethasone, hydrocortisone); however, ulcerative proctitis can be very stubborn, and often returns quickly when drugs are withdrawn. Significant corticosteroid is absorbed from the inflamed rectum, producing unwanted systemic effects.

Chronic use of rectal steroid treatments therefore should be avoided. An oral 5-ASA drug such as mesalamine or sulfasalazine may be used for longer periods to maintain a remission (Chapter 20).

MILD ULCERATIVE COLITIS

Mild ulcerative colitis has few systemic symptoms such as fever, weight loss, and anemia. Tiny and minimally bleeding ulcers are seen by sigmoidoscopy and are usually confined to the left colon. Such a mild attack may be treated by one of the 5-ASA compounds (Chapter 20). Sulfasalazine, the original 5-ASA drug, may be given in a dose of two 500-milligram tablets four times a day, and in those who can tolerate it, 8 or even 12 grams per day. Enteric-coated tablets make it easier for those who suffer nausea or indigestion from the drug. Because this drug is occasionally used for arthritis, it may be desirable when the joints are affected as an extraintestinal manifestation of IBD (Chapter 16).

It is probable, though, that most new patients with colitis will be treated with one of the newer 5-ASA drugs. As many as a third of people cannot tolerate sulfasalazine because of the side-effects, which are largely attributable to the sulfonamide component of the drug. In the newer 5-ASA drugs, the 5-ASA is not coupled with a sulfonamide, thus eliminating many of the undesirable effects (Chapter 20).

The 5-ASA in sulfasalazine is released from the sulfonamide in the colon by bacteria (see Figure 20-1). The newer compounds modify or replace this colon delivery system. Olsalazine (Dipentum) is a double 5-ASA molecule joined by a diazo bond similar to that of sulfasalazine (see Figure 20-2). It appears to be especially effective in left-sided colitis, but is costly and may cause diarrhea. Mesalamine (Asacol, Salofalk, Mesasal, Pentasa) is 5-ASA in capsules designed to release the drug in the lower gut, triggered by the higher pH found there (see Table 20-1). The greatest experience is with Asacol, which may be taken in a dose of 4.8 grams per day (twelve 400-milligram capsules), but 3.2 grams is more common. Belief in the efficacy of these new drugs is largely extrapolated from the large experience with sulfasalazine, although there are some encouraging trials. Rarely, one encounters a patient whose diarrhea paradoxically worsens on 5-ASA. When the drug is stopped, improvement occurs.

If the disease is confined to the rectosigmoid, topical therapy may be practical. Four-gram 5-ASA enemas (Salofalk) achieve results as good as or better than steroid enemas. They are employed once or twice daily, and as a rule of thumb, they should be continued a week after the bleeding ceases to ensure healing. When 5-ASA enemas fail or are not tolerated, steroid enemas may be used.

Most mild attacks can be managed on an ambulatory basis with little interference with diet or activity; however, some common-sense rules apply. One should avoid drugs that are known to irritate the colon. These include laxatives and the nonsteroidal antiinflammatory drugs (NSAIDs) used in arthritis. Broad-spectrum antibiotics, such as ampicillin, alter the gut flora and encourage overgrowth of toxin-producing organisms that cause antibiotic-associated colitis. Caffeine and the laxative artificial sweeteners found in diet gum should be avoided. The diet should be adequate: three meals a day with regular meat protein and fresh vegetables (Chapter 25). Avoid any food previously known to upset the gut. If unable to tolerate milk, one should exclude it (see lactose intolerance, Chapter 25). Normal activity is permitted, but fatigue or excessive stress is best avoided. Most mild attacks improve promptly; nevertheless, an attack may unexpectedly worsen, so vigilance is required.

MODERATE ULCERATIVE COLITIS

Here the disease is more active, with much rectal bleeding and pus, fever, and some weight loss. At sigmoidoscopy the physician sees actively bleeding ulcers, and the disease often extends beyond the splenic flexure. Such an attack usually requires that the patient stay home from work or school. Appetite may be poor, and eating is followed by yet more diarrhea. In a well-nourished patient, a clear fluid diet will keep him or her hydrated for a few days until improvement begins to occur. Oral 5-ASA compounds are often insufficient treatment for such an attack. If the disease is confined to the rectosigmoid, 5-ASA or steroid enemas may be tried. There are several steroid enemas available [betamethasone 5 milligrams; hydrocortisone, 100 milligrams; hydrocortisone acetate (Cortifoam) containing approximately 1 gram hydrocortisone; etc]. A therapeutic enema should be retained as high and as long as possible. Such treatment is difficult if the patient suffers much urgency or tenesmus (painful urge to defecate).

In most cases of moderately severe ulcerative colitis, oral prednisone is the drug of choice (see Steroids, Chapter 21). The usual starting dose is 40 milligrams per day. If the patient can tolerate it, eight 5-milligram tablets may be taken as a single morning dose. Many patients experience heartburn, however, and do better when fractions of the dose are given in a two-times- or four-times-daily routine. In children, alternate-day treatment is sometimes employed to minimize suppression of natural cortisone secretion by the adrenal glands. Once a remission is achieved, the dose must be reduced stepwise to the lowest dose that controls the disease. Optimally that dose should eventually be zero. Common instructions are as follows: Reduce the dose at weekly intervals to 30, 25, 20, 17.5, 15, 12.5, 10, 7.5, 5, 2.5 milligrams, and then discontinue the drug. If symptoms return while tapering, return to the last effective dose and call the physician. Maintenance at this level may be necessary for a while, but one should always test the possibility of reducing the drug, because the natural tendency of the disease is to remit. In view of the potential side-effects of steroids, the aim should be to quit the drug when it is not required. When this is achieved, a prophylactic dose of 5-ASA is started.

Symptomatic therapy should be kept to a minimum. When diarrhea is especially troublesome, a small dose of loperamide (Imodium), one or two tablets, may be given cautiously. Regular dosage may paralyze the bowel and precipitate a toxic megacolon. Pain relief is also tricky. Acetaminophen (Tylenol) is safe, but codeine and other narcotics constipate the bowel and risk drug dependency.

SEVERE ULCERATIVE COLITIS

A severe attack of ulcerative colitis is characterized by fever; feeling unwell, even prostration; anemia; loss of appetite and weight; and profuse bloody diarrhea, often with tenesmus. The sigmoidoscopic picture is of extensive ulceration and much pus and blood, and the disease often extends to the cecum. There is risk of the life-threatening complications discussed in the next chapter.

A person with such an attack should be admitted to a hospital. Bed rest with bathroom privileges is often prescribed, but some exercise, especially of the legs, is important to prevent clotting in the veins (thrombophlebitis). Initially nothing is taken by mouth, because many believe a period of gut rest is helpful. At least, such diet restriction reduces the diarrhea and improves morale. If blood loss has been great, and the anemia is severe, a blood transfusion may be required. Fluid and salt needs may be supplied by intravenous administration of sodium and potassium. Glucose in the intravenous solution provides a few calories; however, it will soon be necessary to eat. Nourishment is graded according to the patient's tolerance by adding first clear fluids, then full fluids, soft diet, and so forth. Sometimes an elemental diet is employed. Such a diet consists of amino acids, glucose, and medium-chain fatty acids, which bypass digestion and are absorbed in the small intestine, leaving little residue for the colon (Chapter 25).

Oral 5-ASA is unlikely to be effective in severe colitis. Treatment enemas or suppositories often cannot be retained. Therefore methylprednisolone (Solu-Medrol) or its equivalent is given intravenously in a dose of 20 milligrams every 8 or 12 hours. Oral prednisone is substituted when eating is resumed. Some physicians advocate hydrocortisone or adrenocorticotropin (ACTH), a pituitary hormone that stimulates the adrenal gland to release cortisone. These are not commonly used now (Chapter 21). The former causes more salt retention and swelling than does prednisone, and the use of ACTH presumes that the adrenal gland is functioning normally. This may not be the case if steroids have been used previously.

It may take 2 or 3 weeks for signs of improvement to occur.

Once the patient is eating normally, he or she may be discharged on oral prednisone with instructions to decrease the drug in the manner described previously. Delay or failure to improve should invite a surgical consultation, in anticipation of a possible colectomy. In the event of such a delay in recovery, nutrition becomes critically important (Chapter 25). If an elemental diet cannot be tolerated, intravenous feeding [total parenteral nutrition (TPN)] may be required. Surgery should not be postponed unduly (Chapter 26).

Antidiarrheal agents that may be cautiously given in mild disease are best avoided here. Codeine, diphenoxylate, or loperamide all relax the gut muscle. Superimposed on the toxic effects of the disease, these drugs may paralyze the colon and precipitate a toxic megacolon. Painkillers may be given for short periods as described previously. Demerol is the preferred narcotic, as it has the least constipating effect.

The need to document progress may pose a dilemma. A gentle sigmoidoscopy confined to the rectum, without preparation and with minimal air, may provide the necessary information. Colonoscopy or barium enema are contraindicated and even dangerous if the colon is severely inflamed. Precise knowledge of the extent of the disease in a patient severely ill with colitis is academic, because it will not alter the treatment.

MAINTENANCE AND PROPHYLAXIS

Maintenance and prophylaxis are not the same. The former is continued treatment of active disease over the time required to control continuing manifestations of the disease. Sometimes colitis may grumble on for weeks or months, requiring ongoing steroid therapy. Usually the disease eventually remits, and in that event, one should not miss the opportunity to discontinue the drug, even if the steroid-free interlude is short lived. Failure of the disease to remit, and the resulting steroid dependence, is an indication for surgery.

Prophylaxis applies to colitis in remission. When the remission is secure, and active treatment is discontinued, a small dose of a

5-ASA compound is effective in reducing recurrent attacks. Sulfasalazine was validated for this purpose 30 years ago. Olsalazine appears to be as effective as sulfasalazine. Asacol and the other 5-ASA compounds of the mesalamine group may be less effective in left-colon colitis, perhaps because the 5-ASA is released higher up in the bowel. The recommended doses are sulfasalazine, 500 milligrams four times a day; olsalazine, 500 milligrams four times a day; or Asacol, 400 milligrams three or four times a day. The choice may ultimately be dictated by cost (see Table 20-2). If no attack occurs for several years on such a prophylactic dose, the drug may be discontinued.

SUMMARY

Treatment of ulcerative colitis must be graded according to the severity and extent of the attack. Mild disease may be managed with a therapeutic dose of a 5-ASA preparation. If only the rectum or rectosigmoid is involved, local treatment is provided by 5-ASA suppositories or enemas. Once the diagnosis is secure, more moderate disease may require steroid treatment, either oral prednisone or, in the case of rectosigmoid disease, steroid enemas. Rest, fluids, and sometimes antidiarrhea drugs permit ambulatory treatment. More severe disease will require admission to a hospital, with intravenous fluid, salts, and methylprednisolone sodium succinate (Solu-Medrol) administration. Careful surveillance is important, because failure to respond necessitates colectomy if complications are to be avoided. As improvement occurs, the prednisone should be withdrawn stepwise, seeking the lowest dose of the drug that controls the disease, which should eventually be nil. Failure to establish a remission sufficient to permit cessation of the steroid within a reasonable period is an indication for colectomy. Once remission is achieved, the prophylactic use of low-dose 5-ASA will reduce the number of recurrent attacks.

CHAPTER TEN

Ulcerative Colitis
Complications

The manifestations of ulcerative colitis are disabling enough. The inflamed mucosa produces local and systemic effects, which themselves compromise an individual's ability to function. Additional troubles in the form of complications sometimes add to this disability. These occur when the disease is severe, or long standing, or extends beyond the colon mucosa. There are two groups of ulcerative colitis complications: those due to progression of the disease itself, such as toxic megacolon, anemia, or cancer; and those due to associated diseases, such as sclerosing cholangitis of rheumatoid spondylitis. The latter are called extraintestinal manifestations of ulcerative colitis. These are similar in Crohn's disease, and will be discussed in a Chapter 16. As if these disease complications were not enough, the unwanted effects of therapy add to the burden (Chapters 20 to 23). Here we concern ourselves with the complications of the colonic mucosal inflammation itself.

LIFE-THREATENING COMPLICATIONS

The serious complications of ulcerative colitis may occur at any time in the course of the disease. There may be a progression from fulminant colitis through toxic megacolon to perforation, but each may occur apparently de novo as well. They imply extension of the inflammatory process beyond the colon mucosa and submucosa. When these complications occur with the first attack, the diagnosis may be difficult, especially in the elderly. Other intestinal diseases such as diverticulitis, ischemic colitis, appendicitis, or even a perforated peptic ulcer are more likely in old people and may present clinical features similar to those of complicated colitis. In ulcerative colitis, whatever the complications, discovery of the characteristically inflamed rectal mucosa through the sigmoido- scope is the key to the diagnosis. When ulcerative colitis is known to exist, the diagnosis of complications may be easier. Even long- standing, nonsystemic ulcerative proctitis may suddenly progress through more extensive colitis to one of its serious sequelae.

Despite the need for vigilance, patients should be reassured that most people with ulcerative colitis will acquire none of these complications. Furthermore, the risk may be reduced with good medical care and judicious surgery.

Fulminant Colitis

Fortunately, fewer than 5 percent of ulcerative colitis patients ever develop fulminant colitis. Some clinicians would rather call it a severe degree of colitis, and not a complication at all. It is a complication, however, in the sense that it is a life-threatening emergency, and it implies impending toxic megacolon or perfora- tion. Prevention, or at least early recognition, of each of these complications is necessary, if lives are not to be lost.

Patients with fulminant colitis are very ill. Diarrhea and hemor- rhage produce severe dehydration, salt loss, and anemia, which may progress to shock. The toxic systemic effects of the severe inflammation produce a fever of up to 40 degrees centigrade (104 degrees Fahrenheit), and extreme prostration. The pulse is rapid, blood pressure is low, and skin is dry, toneless, and pallid. The abdomen is tender and tense, and there may be evidence of inflammation extending to the serosal or peritoneal layer of the gut. Confusion, delirium, even unconsciousness may intervene. Death occurs unless urgent resuscitation is employed.

The white blood cell and platelet counts are usually high, and hemoglobin and albumin (blood protein) may be low. Blood clotting may be impaired. Minerals such as sodium and potassium may be depleted. Normal at first, serial abdominal plain films may detect a dilating (expanding) colon (Figure 10-1). Barium enema and colonoscopy are dangerous in this setting, because they may precipitate megacolon or perforation. Sigmoidoscopy may be essential to confirm the diagnosis of ulcerative colitis. Only the rectosigmoid need be studied, and air insufflation should be minimal.

A patient with fulminant disease should be in the hospital with no oral intake and with intravenous therapy and excellent nursing care. Resuscitation includes an intravenous solution containing sodium and potassium. Blood loss is treated by transfusions, and blood clotting is optimized. In a new case, intravenous steroids are administered [methylprednisolone (Solu-Medrol) 20 milligrams twice or three times daily]. Many patients slipping into fulminant colitis are already on this treatment, however, and must be deemed treatment failures.

A surgeon should be consulted. Even those patients who achieve remission may require surgery later. It is best to try to stabilize the disease with medical therapy and operate when the patient's condition improves. This is not, however, always an option, and deterioration or failure to improve should trigger prompt surgery, if toxic megacolon, perforation, or even death are to be avoided. Such consequences should not occur with modern medicine and surgery.

Toxic Megacolon

This, the most dramatic of all colitis complications, occurs in fewer than 1 percent of cases, and seems more likely in the young or newly diagnosed. If fulminant colitis is treated with dispatch, this

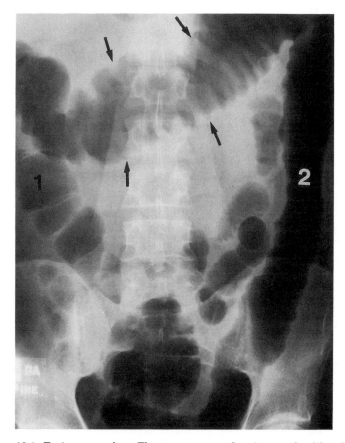

Figure 10-1. Toxic megacolon. The transverse colon is greatly dilated and threatens to burst (arrows). Notice the lack of haustral features in the colon margins. Compare with Figure 8-1. The ascending colon (1) is normal. The descending colon (2) has an irregular pattern due to ulcers and submucosal edema.

complication should be rare. Toxic megacolon (Figure 10-1) is not unique to ulcerative colitis. It may also complicate colitis due to shigella or salmonella, and occasionally Crohn's colitis.

This complication is largely preventable. Patients admitted to the hospital with severe, extensive colitis should have daily girth measurements and abdominal plain films until they improve. As toxic megacolon develops, the transverse colon dilates. In this complication, the inflammation advances from its stronghold in the mucosa to invade the muscularis and serosa. This and the patient's general toxicity paralyze the colon, which may then distend to the point of bursting. For this reason, in severe disease, it is unwise to employ drugs to treat severe diarrhea and cramps. These include opiate or anticholinergic drugs, which reduce colon contractions and may further reduce colon muscle tone. As in infectious colitis, diarrhea, like sneezing, is a defense mechanism to rid the gut of unwanted organisms and tissue debris. Even in mild colitis, anti-diarrhea agents must therefore be used with caution.

Toxic megacolon displays the features of fulminant colitis; however, the flaccid muscles of the colon permit it to dilate and fill with air and fluid. The abdomen becomes distended, painful, and tender, and a supine plain abdominal x-ray will show a dilated, air-filled transverse colon (Figure 10-1). A segment measuring more than 6 centimeters in diameter is considered critical. The remainder of the colon is also dilated, but is filled with fluid so that it may not show on the plain film. The diarrhea and bleeding may seem to subside. This apparent paradox does not mean improvement, but rather that blood and fecal fluid are retained in the colon. The distended, rigid abdomen may produce a tympanitic sound when tapped with the examining finger, and no bowel sounds are heard.

Rarely a previously normal colon may dilate following surgery or severe injury. This is a form of pseudo-obstruction, sometimes called *Ogilvie's syndrome*, and the right colon may dilate to an alarming degree, threatening perforation. Toxic megacolon may be suspected in such cases, but sigmoidoscopic examination of the rectosigmoid quickly rules out colitis. Often this process may be reversed by decompression of the cecum through a colonoscope. This is not an option in toxic megacolon.

Toxic megacolon is a surgical emergency. Perforation of the

bowel is imminent, and medical means cannot be expected to reverse the process. Antibiotics should be administered as one prepares for surgery. Cautious attempts to decompress the colon are only temporary measures. A nasogastric tube, complete with suction, reduces the contribution of swallowed air. A carefully placed rectal tube may decompress the rectum. Although a long tube passed via the stomach and small gut into the cecum may produce a temporary reprieve, the technique is difficult, and should not be employed as a means to delay surgery. The mortality of this complication is 30 percent, and even among those who survive the crisis without surgery, most eventually require proctocolectomy. With modern operative techniques, delayed colectomy can seldom be justified.

Perforation

Colon perforation (Figure 10-2) as a result of progression through fulminant colitis or toxic megacolon is a medical failure. Rarely, perforation may occur in the first severe attack without the usual antecedents. It might occur during periods of increased luminal pressure, such as during colonoscopy or barium enema, and these procedures should be avoided in acute colitis. In these unexpected cases, there may be a very local extension of the inflammation through the muscle layer of the bowel.

Early recognition of such an event is crucial. Usually sudden abdominal pain, fever, toxicity, and the physical signs of an acute (surgical) abdomen betray the diagnosis; however, such features may be muted somewhat by the antiinflammatory effects of adrenocorticoid (steroid) therapy. This is the gravest complication of ulcerative colitis, and immediate, life-saving surgery is required.

Massive Hemorrhage

Bleeding is a common, virtually universal feature of ulcerative colitis. Generally the degree of blood loss varies with the extent of the disease and the severity of the colonic ulceration. Rarely,

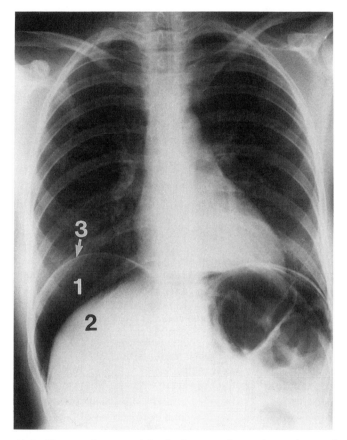

Figure 10-2. Chest and upper abdominal x-ray of a patient whose colon has perforated as a result of severe ulcerative colitis. Note the air (1) that is free in the abdominal cavity, lying outside the intestines between the liver (2) and diaphragm (3). This x-ray was taken with the patient upright.

bleeding may be sudden, profound, and life threatening. The very ill colitis sufferer, who may already be anemic from chronic blood loss or marrow suppression, can ill afford a massive loss of blood. Falling blood pressure and rapid pulse mark the body's attempt to compensate for the depleted blood volume, and shock may ensue, if vigorous transfusions are not employed to prevent it. Any defect in blood coagulation should be corrected. Usually, such medical means control the situation, but, occasionally colectomy is needed to prevent a fatal hemorrhage.

CHRONIC DISABLING COMPLICATIONS

Anemia

Red blood cells contain a red pigment called hemoglobin, which carries oxygen from the lungs to the tissues. Chronic loss of blood and toxic depression of bone marrow production of new red cells result in a reduced red cell population in the blood. This is called anemia. Other measures of the degree of anemia are the hemoglobin and the hematocrit (red cell volume). Anemia is usually tolerated well in the young, but the impaired oxygen-carrying capacity of hemoglobin-poor anemic blood increases the risk of cardiac ischemia (angina), breathlessness, and stroke in the elderly.

As blood is lost from the veins and arteries, fluid from the tissues enters these vessels to make up the lost volume. The resulting dilution of the red cells causes the hemoglobin and hematocrit to fail. As the bone marrow steps up production of red cells, it consumes iron, an essential component of hemoglobin. The inevitable iron deficiency impairs the marrow's ability to keep up. In apparent frustration, it produces small, hemoglobin-poor cells, identified by direct examination of the blood. This condition is called a *microcytic, hypochromic anemia*. Oral administration of iron becomes necessary (Chapter 25). Cardiac patients may require a transfusion of red cells to boost oxygen-carrying capacity. Bone marrow depression due to the general toxicity of the disease impairs the usual compensatory mechanisms, so that even when bleeding is controlled, and iron is restored, there remains an *anemia of chronic disease*.

Other factors contribute to the anemia. Poor diet may lead to folic acid deficiency. Found in most fruits, vegetables and meats, this B vitamin is, like iron, an essential factor in the manufacture of hemoglobin, the oxygen-carrying pigment of red cells. Folate deficiency induces the marrow to produce immature, large (macrocytic) cells. Anemia may be further compounded by increased red cell destruction in the spleen and other tissues. Such *hemolysis* may be an unwanted effect of drugs such as sulfasalazine.

Malnutrition

Digestion and absorption of nutrients occur mainly in the small intestine, whose function should be unimpaired in ulcerative colitis. This contrasts with small-bowel Crohn's disease, in which weight loss and other nutritional consequences are prominent. Nevertheless, in severe ulcerative colitis, poor oral intake due to loss of appetite or "bowel rest" combines with losses from, and energy consumption by, the inflamed colon to malnourish the patient (see Chapter 25).

Protein losses are particularly important. Albumin is lost through the inflamed mucosa and not adequately replaced. Albumin provides the most important intravascular osmotic force, so a very low blood albumin may permit fluid to leak into the tissues. This is manifested by swelling (edema) of dependent parts such as the ankles. To compensate, protein is recruited from muscle, leading to muscle wasting. Similar sequences produce net loss of carbohydrate (starch, sugar) and fat, the principal sources of energy. Lassitude and weight loss ensue.

Poor food intake may produce vitamin and mineral deficiencies as well. The B vitamins are particularly vulnerable, especially folic acid. Vitamin K deficiency may impair the blood's ability to clot, an important factor when the colon weeps blood. The *prothrombin time* measures this effect.

Fluid, salt, and vitamin deficiencies can be prevented or corrected, even in severe disease, by judicious intravenous replacement. Protein and calorie malnutrition is less easily handled. Because the severely ill patient cannot eat, weight loss and wasting may become serious, provoking colectomy. The use of elemental or defined diets, or total intravenous nutrition is discussed in Chapter 25.

Growth Retardation

The issues discussed in the previous section are poignantly apparent in adolescents. Here the growing body's needs for protein for muscle, calcium for bone, and iron for blood outstrip the meager supplies remaining after the demands of inflammation are satisfied. Stature becomes retarded in 5 to 10 percent of children with ulcerative colitis. Growth areas at each end of a bone are called epiphyses. When growth of a particular bone is complete, its epiphyses fuse, permitting no further growth. Determined largely by one's biological clock, the fusions occur at certain ages, whether the bone has grown enough, or not; thus, growth delayed by inflammatory bowel disease (IBD) beyond the date of fusion is irredeemable. Like stature, secondary sexual characteristics are retarded. Add these personal catastrophes to the adolescent's need to cope with diarrhea, disability, and the effects of prednisone, and severe psychologic consequences seem inevitable. Early colectomy may be the only recourse.

Anorectal Complications

Anal fistula, fissure, and abscess are far less likely in ulcerative colitis than in Crohn's disease, and are discussed in that section. Urgency and incontinence are common. In acute disease, the inflamed rectum is hypersensitive and overreacts to even small amounts of stool. In chronic disease, the colon and rectum become narrow, a rigid tube without the normal storage function (Figure 10-3). Both processes are aggravated by the constant arrival of a large volume of liquid stool, which contrives to overwhelm the anal

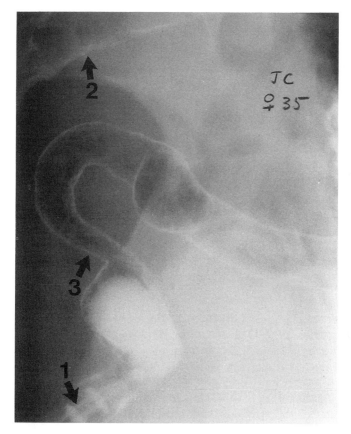

Figure 10-3. Lateral view of a barium-filled rectum of a patient with ulcerative colitis: (1) barium delivery catheter; (2) sacrum or tail bone; (3) narrowed, ulcerated, rigid rectum and lower sigmoid. Weeping blood and fluid, this rectum has no storage capacity. Even when the colitis is in remission, this useless, scarred rectum and sigmoid fails to permit fecal storage and normal, controlled defecation.

sphincter. The sufferer dare not stray far from the bathroom lest he or she suffer an accident. In severe cases of rectal inflammation, the urge to defecate becomes painful (tenesmus), or straining causes rectal tissue to protrude through the anus (rectal prolapse).

Increased anal traffic and vigorous wiping cause troublesome excoriations of the skin around the anus. Itching and a sense of soiling motivate the sufferer to scrub, indeed polish, the area. Damage to nerve endings in the skin relieves the itch; however, gratification is fleeting. The nerve endings soon recover, setting in motion the itch–scratch cycle. Relief depends largely on control of the diarrhea, but cleansing with a gentle water flow and a pat dry with a lint-free cloth help. Tucs, or Wet Ones are portable substitutes. One must resist the temptation to scratch. Toilet paper is traumatizing, and bits of paper trapped in the anal crevices may irritate. Ointments and creams, especially those containing a local anesthetic, may be allergenic, may impair the anal seal, or may harbor bacteria. A very light application of a cortisone-bearing cream may help.

Colon Stricture

Repeated, severe attacks of ulcerative colitis may scar and constrict the colon. The resulting stricture (Figure 10-4) is usually asymptomatic, discovered incidentally by colonoscopy or barium enema. Rarely it may obstruct the colon, but the principal cause for concern is its resemblance to colon cancer. The benign stricture has tapered ends rather than a shouldering effect, as in cancer, but even experienced endoscopists and radiologists are seldom willing to declare a stricture noncancerous. Multiple cancer-free biopsies of the mucosa lining the stricture may be reassuring, but only with examination of the complete colectomy specimen can one be certain.

COLON CANCER

Those whose ulcerative colitis has been present for a decade or longer are increasingly liable to malignant change (Figure 10-5) in

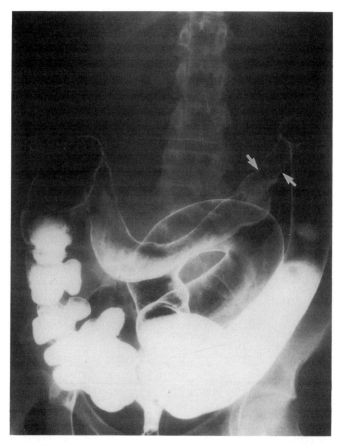

Figure 10-4. Stricture of the transverse colon near the splenic flexure. This patient, a 25-year-old woman, had ulcerative colitis since age 8. Because of concern that the stricture might be a carcinoma, she underwent colectomy. No cancer was found.

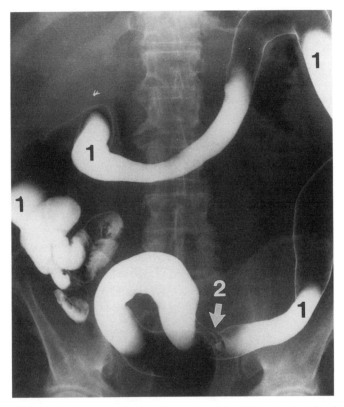

Figure 10-5. Barium enema showing the entire colon (1) involved with advanced ulcerative colitis. Note the shortened, narrowed, and featureless colon. Haustra are absent. Compare to Figure 27-9. The irregular shadow (2) in the sigmoid colon indicates complicating colon cancer.

the colon mucosa. The exact risk is controversial, but it is certainly greater with pancolitis, long duration, and onset in youth. Thus after 10 years of disease, most pundits recommend periodic surveillance of the colon mucosa through colonoscopy and biopsy. The presence of colon epithelial dysplasia is a harbinger of cancer. In some centers, early colectomy is practiced in high-risk patients, based on the thesis that dysplasia provides insufficient warning. This controversial topic is discussed further in Chapters 17 and 26.

PSYCHOLOGICAL COMPLICATIONS

Young people have difficulty coping with a disease that sets them aside from their peers. The psychologic features are sometimes very pronounced. In the 1930s, Engel implicated psychologic disturbances in the causation of ulcerative colitis. According to psychosomatic theory, psychologic factors expose colitis in one biologically susceptible to the disease. Medical observers have usually taken the opposite position. Ill, growth-retarded, steroid-disfigured youths unable to participate in activity far from a toilet are subject to psychologic trauma undreamt of by their peers. These important gut reactions are explored further in Chapter 18.

SUMMARY

Life-threatening complications of ulcerative colitis include fulminant colitis, toxic megacolon, perforation, and massive hemorrhage. Good medical care, alertness to these complications, and timely surgery should prevent them, and deaths should be rare. Chronic complications include anemia, nutritional deficiencies, growth retardation, anorectal disease, and stricture. Malignant and psychologic complications require whole chapters in Part 4.

PART THREE

Crohn's Disease

CHAPTER ELEVEN

Crohn's Disease
Pathology and Pathogenesis

The cases gave the impression that they were probably tuberculosis, and yet from the uniform character of the affection it evidently is not so. The affected bowel gives the smoothness of an eel in a state of rigor mortis, and the glands, though enlarged are evidently not caseous.

T. K. Dalziel, 1913

Crohn's disease shares many characteristics with ulcerative colitis. They have a common epidemiology and relapsing nature, are of unknown case, share extraintestinal complications, and have a similar response to some drugs. When disease is confined to the colon, differentiation is initially unimportant, because drug and diet recommendations are the same. This is fortunate; in 10 to 20 percent of instances, even skilled clinicians and pathologists are unable to differentiate between the two. However, the long-term outlook, the opportunities for drug and surgical management, the quality of life, and the complications are much different in Crohn's disease from those in ulcerative colitis.

DIFFERENCES FROM ULCERATIVE COLITIS

The cause of both diseases is unknown, so the differences are best explained by pathology (Table 11-1). Whereas ulcerative colitis is confined to the colon, Crohn's disease may involve any segment of the gut. Unlike that in ulcerative colitis, surgical extirpation of the affected bowel offers no cure, and recurrences are the rule. Crohn's disease affects all layers of the gut. This feature, even when the disease is confined to the colon, is the basis of the very different set of symptoms and complications found in that disease compared to colitis. Whereas the latter is characterized by diarrhea and bleeding, the thickened gut wall of Crohn's disease may narrow and obstruct the lumen, or a deep ulcer may extend beyond the serosa to cause an abscess or fistula. Although the rectum is almost always involved in ulcerative colitis, and extends in a continuum to a variable extent proximally (nearer the cecum), Crohn's disease will often spare the rectum, and is discontinuous, with "skip" areas of normal gut bracketing areas of disease.

In colorectal disease, it may be very difficult, short of surgery, to distinguish ulcerative colitis from Crohn's colitis. The appearance of the mucosa may be similar in both diseases. Rectal biopsy through a sigmoidoscope provides only mucosal tissue, and may also fail to differentiate between the two diseases. Patchy involve-

TABLE 11-1
Pathology of Crohn's Diesease and Ulcerative Colitis

Crohn's disease	Ulcerative colitis
• All gut layers	• Mucosa
• Whole gut	• Colon
• Discontinuous, rectal sparing	• Continuous from anus
• Granuloma	• Crypt abscess
• Obstruction, fistula	• Diarrhea, bleeding
• Abdominal mass	• No abdominal mass
• Less cancer risk	• Colon cancer risk

ment, deep, irregular ulcers, and heaped-up mucosa suggest Crohn's disease to the endoscopist, but the initial clinical diagnosis is often *indeterminate* colitis. When the clinician is uncertain, the pathologist is seldom able to settle the matter from a mucosal biopsy. Crypt abscesses and pseudopolyp formation suggest ulcerative colitis, and patchy involvement, granulomas, and fistulas are more common features of Crohn's disease. None of these is specific for either. Crohn's disease is associated with an increased incidence of bowel cancer, but the risk is much less than that found in ulcerative colitis. Thus, in colitis, surgery might be considered to be both curative and a cancer prophylaxis. Neither consideration applies in Crohn's disease, in which the surgical role is to treat complications of the disease.

PATHOLOGY

Crohn's disease may affect any level of the gut. Only the small bowel is involved in one fourth of cases, only the colon in about one fifth of cases, and the ileocecal region in about one half. The remaining cases involve disease of the anus, the duodenum, the stomach, or the esophagus. Any combination is, of course, possible. The inflammatory process is similar at all levels of affected gut, but symptoms differ depending on the site of involvement, the severity and disturbance of function at that site, and the narrowness of the lumen. The terminal ileum is the most commonly affected segment, and the cecum is usually involved as well. There may be skip areas in the small bowel or left colon. Despite the observation that rectal involvement suggests ulcerative colitis, it also occurs in more than 50 percent of cases of colonic Crohn's. The entire colon is involved in one fourth of cases of Crohn's colitis, and skip areas within the colon are seen in another fourth.

Early lesions of Crohn's disease appear to the sigmoidoscopist as small, shallow, discrete ulcers. Adjacent to such an ulcer, a granuloma may be found in a biopsy (see the following). The tiny ulcers are usually asymptomatic, but may tip off the observer that there is trouble higher up. Similar lesions appear as cold sores in the mouth and throat, and are called *aphthous ulcers*. More severe disease may appear as erythema, with blood, pus, friability, and tiny ulcers similar to those of ulcerative colitis.

Later a combination of deep ulcers and swollen mucosa and submucosa generates a lumpy, paved quality to the luminal surface of the gut (Figure 11-1). On x-ray, this is described as a "cobblestone" appearance (see Figure 12-1). At other sites the ulcers may be deep, and tend to lie in the axis of the bowel. The ulcers may be undermined, and cast a "collarbutton" silhouette in a barium contrast x-ray. Between the diseased areas there may be relatively normal bowel.

Although the inflammation involves all layers of the gut, it is most marked in the submucosa, which becomes choked with

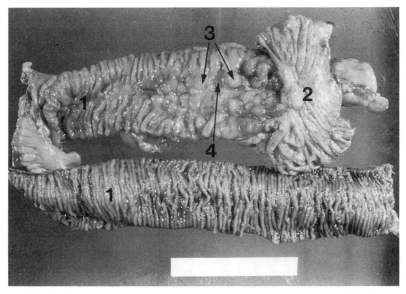

Figure 11-1. Surgically removed terminal ileum (1) and cecum (2). Note the raised, smooth areas in the ileum near the ileocecal valve (3). These produce a pavement quality or "cobblestone" effect on barium contrast x-ray (see Figure 12-1). Ulcers lie between the cobblestones (4).

chronic inflammatory cells (lymphocytes, histiocytes, and mono-nuclear cells). Blood and lymph vessels become engorged, and fluid seeps into the tissues (edema). Later fibrous tissue participates in the repair process, which causes scarring. The result is a thickened, rubbery bowel wall and disruption of the normal tissues, eventually beyond recognition (see Dalziel's description at the beginning of this chapter). Infiltration of acute inflammatory cells (polymorpho-nuclear leukocytes) and the formation of crypt abscesses are less common than in ulcerative colitis. The tissue destruction breeds ulcers, which may coalesce and penetrate deeply through the submucosa. As the ulcers deepen, they burrow through the serosa to cause abscesses or fistulas into skin or other organs (Figure 11-2).

One reason for the long delay in the recognition of Crohn's disease was its similarity, noted by Dalziel, to intestinal tuber-culosis. Like Crohn's, tuberculosis has a predilection for the termi-nal ileum, and has a tendency to produce granulomas. Fortunately, intestinal tuberculosis is seldom encountered in modern indus-trialized countries. Details of the nature of granulomas are found in textbooks of pathology. For our purposes, a granuloma may be described as a discrete microscopic collection of chronic inflamma-tory cells, including multinucleated *giant* cells and large *epithelioid* cells (Figure 11-3). They are found in several chronic infections, such as tuberculosis, and in chronic inflammations of unknown cause, such as sarcoidosis or Crohn's disease. In the former, the granu-lomas have a core of destroyed tissue called *caseation*. The granu-lomas of Crohn's disease are said to be noncaseating. The presence of granulomas has inspired the notion that chronic infection by an organism similar to the tubercle bacillus (*Mycobacterium*) is respons-ible for Crohn's disease. Despite studies of many candidate organ-isms, and even animal models of mycobacterial infection, no organism has a proven association with Crohn's. Granulomas are found not only in the walls of resected specimens, but also in lymph nodes, peritoneum, and even the liver. Occasionally, one may discover a granuloma on a rectal biopsy, especially in early lesions; however, in many cases granulomas are never found, even at surgery. These curious lesions, therefore, are neither sensitive nor specific indicators of Crohn's disease.

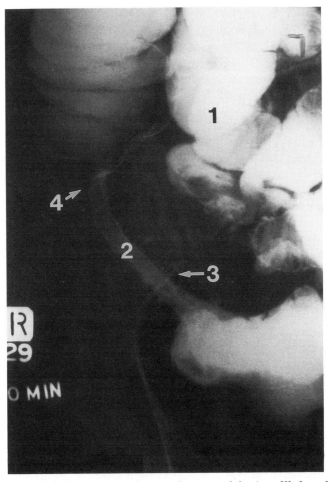

Figure 11-2. Small-bowel enema. Compared to normal, barium-filled small bowel
(1), the terminal ileum (2) is narrowed, and the space surrounding this segment
indicates a greatly thickened gut wall. Note the deep, barium-filled ulcers or
fissures extending through the wall at right angles to the gut lumen (3). When
these penetrate beyond the wall, fistulas develop. This patient had a previous
ileocecal resection, and this x-ray represents a recurrence, typically proximal to
the anastomosis (4).

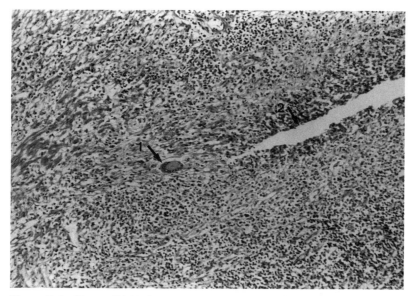

Figure 11-3. Giant cell (1) indicating a granuloma in the gut wall of a patient with Crohn's disease. A collection of giant and epithelioid cells is suggestive, but not diagnostic, of Crohn's. Note the deep fissure (2) adjacent to the granuloma.

PATHOGENESIS

The disease is clinically featured by symptoms that resemble those of ulcerative colitis, namely, fever, diarrhoea, and emaciation, leading eventually to an obstruction of the small intestine; the constant occurrence of a mass in the right iliac fossa usually requires surgical intervention (resection). The terminal ileum is alone involved. The process begins abruptly at and involves the ileocecal valve in its maximal intensity, tapering off gradually as it ascends the ileum for from 8 to 12 inches (20 to 30 cm.). The familiar fistulas lead usually to segments of colon, forming small tracts communicating with the lumen of the large intestine; occasionally the abdominal wall, anteriorly, is the site of one or more of these fistulous tracts.

B. B. Crohn, L. Ginsberg, and G. D. Oppenheimer, 1932

The clinical manifestations of Crohn's disease depend on the site(s) of the disease in the gut, the extent and severity of inflammation, the degree of gut narrowing, and fistula formation. Small-gut disease is more likely to obstruct, causing abdominal pain, vomiting, and sometimes decreased bowel movements. Colon disease, on the other hand, is more likely to present with the features of colitis: diarrhea, blood, and pus, with abdominal cramps. Extensive and severe inflammation will cause systemic signs, such as fever, malaise, and weight loss. Severe small-bowel involvement may produce poor food intake, malabsorption, and protein loss. Chronic bleeding may combine with a suppressed bone marrow to render the patient anemic. The inflammation is indicated by a high white blood cell count, platelet count, and erythrocyte sedimentation rate (ESR), a low serum protein (albumin), and a low hemoglobin.

Because most nutrients are absorbed in the jejunum, extensive disease there, or surgical removal, may lead to calorie malnutrition and deficiencies in vitamins and minerals. Uniquely, vitamin B_{12} absorption is confined to the terminal ileum, a frequent site of Crohn's disease. Disease or resection of more than 60 centimeters of terminal ileum may cause B_{12} malabsorption. Bile salts are also absorbed in the terminal ileum. Their complicated metabolism is discussed later, but here it should be noted that malabsorbed bile salts cause a *cholerrheic* diarrhea.

Narrowing of the gut sufficient to cause obstruction is more likely to occur in the small intestine. Unable to push food through the narrowed or inactive segment, the gut immediately above the obstruction contracts vigorously, causing abdominal cramps. Eventually this obstructed gut dilates (see Figure 14-1). Also, a fistula may track to the peritoneal (abdominal) cavity, causing an abscess, or to skin, vagina, bladder, and even to another segment of the gut itself (see Figure 14-3).

SUMMARY

Unlike ulcerative colitis, Crohn's disease may affect all levels and all layers of the gut. The chronic inflammation is greatest in the submucosa. Eventually mucosal ulcers appear, which coalesce, undermine, and become very deep, in some cases penetrating the serosa. Heaped-up submucosa, circumscribed by deep ulcers, is responsible for the cobblestone appearance seen on x-rays. Elsewhere, deep, linear ulcers are surrounded by a relatively normal mucosa. Symptoms depend on the site(s), extent, and degree of inflammation, and the range of symptoms is more varied than that of ulcerative colitis. Obstruction occurs when the inflamed segment becomes inactive, or blocks the lumen, usually of the small bowel. An ulcer may become a deep fissure that in turn, becomes a fistula that tracks to an abscess or an adjacent organ.

CHAPTER TWELVE

Crohn's Disease

Symptoms and Diagnosis

. . . most violent colic, causing vomiting and occasionally an escape of
some blood. The bowel becoming exhausted, or the content being
forced through the rigid portion, the patient then would be at rest . . .

T. K. Dalziel, 1913

Crohn's disease has many incarnations. That succinctly described
by Dalziel is due to disease in the small bowel. In contrast, disease
confined to the colon is likely to resemble ulcerative colitis, whereas
perianal or ileocecal Crohn's are different again. Crohn's disease
may present with one of its complications, such as obstruction,
fistula, or abscess. These complications are explained in Chapter 14.
Here we describe the symptoms, signs, and laboratory findings of
the disease according to anatomic site, remembering that in some
patients, more than one site may be involved.

GENERAL SYMPTOMS

Like ulcerative colitis, Crohn's disease is a chronic relapsing
inflammation that may produce systemic or general symptoms.

Chemicals released by the inflammatory cells produce fever. Energy consumption by inflammation and fever produces weight loss and malaise. These, in turn, are aggravated by poor appetite and vomiting. Chronic blood loss, a suppressed bone marrow, and iron or folate deficiencies due to losses and poor diet almost invariably produce anemia. The low hemoglobin and loss of sleep due to symptoms compound the patient's lassitude.

In severe, uncomplicated disease, all the general features described under ulcerative colitis may occur. Protein, fluid, and salt losses can be profound. If the small bowel is involved, the nutritional consequences may dominate the clinical picture, particularly if surgical resection has been necessary.

The psychological consequences are also similar to those of ulcerative colitis, but two circumstances carry an additional impact. First, unlike ulcerative colitis, there is no cure for Crohn's disease. No matter how carefully the lesion is excised, the disease invariably returns. Second, perineal disease in young people may have severe psychosocial repercussions. Despite the fact that reproductive function is ultimately preserved, early, destructive disease near the sexual organs can be a devastating burden.

ILEOCECAL CROHN'S DISEASE

The terminal ileum is the most frequent site of involvement. Usually the cecum is also involved. The characteristic clinical features are abdominal pain and diarrhea. The pain is of two types. The first is due to local inflammation of the outer surface of the gut. In ileocecal Crohn's disease (Figure 12-1), this pain is localized to the right lower quadrant of the abdomen. This area becomes very tender to the touch. The second pain results from the rigid, narrowed lumen that reluctantly permits passage of intestinal contents. The normal gut above the diseased area undergoes repeated, vigorous contractions to force the contents along. The patient interprets this as crampy, or intermittent abdominal pain, usually in the area around the umbilicus. As the disease becomes more obstructive, the normal bowel above dilates, and vomiting may occur.

The diarrhea is usually less severe than that of colitis, because

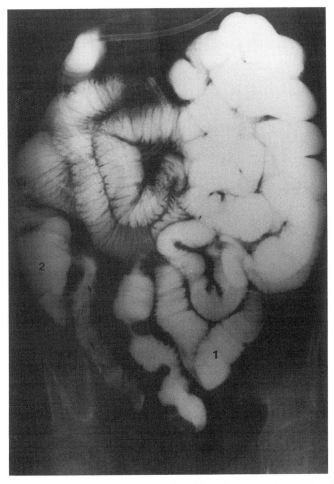

Figure 12-1. Ileocecal Crohn's disease. Small-bowel enema (note tube through which barium was injected) showing disease in the terminal ileum. Arrows point out "cobblestoning." Compare the affected area with normal ileum (1). The cecum (2) appears normal here. Compare also with a normal small-bowel enema (Figure 27-8).

the normal colon is able to salvage excess luminal fluid, and ileal narrowing may slow intestinal transit. Failure of absorption of nutrients and/or bile salts draws fluid into the gut lumen by osmosis. This may increase the fluid load to the colon beyond its ability to absorb. The inflamed gut also exudes protein-rich fluid. Usually the diarrhea is not bloody, but there is chronic, occult blood loss. Rarely a massive bleed due to a ruptured blood vessel may require transfusions or emergency surgery.

The examining physician may first observe marked tenderness over the ileocecal area (right lower quadrant of the abdomen). A thin person may display visible abdominal distention and/or small-bowel peristalsis. Later thickened loops of bowel form a tender lump or mass, which may be felt by the patient or doctor.

The rapidity of onset of these symptoms and signs is highly variable; therefore, clinically the disease may resemble a variety of other conditions. At one extreme, sudden onset of right lower quadrant abdominal pain, cramps, local tenderness, and fever may pose as an acute appendix. In some patients Crohn's disease is first diagnosed by operation for a presumed appendix, but modern ultrasound techniques should make this less common. Occasionally yersinia or campylobacter infections may present in a similar manner. On the other hand, slower onset of diarrhea and cramps with little fever may initially be mistaken for the irritable bowel syndrome. A careful history examination, and blood work should clarify the situation. Symptoms occurring with menses should suggest endometriosis. The development of an abdominal mass above the right groin may make distinction between Crohn's and an appendiceal abscess difficult. Older patients with Crohn's disease and a mass may first be thought to have a tumor such as lymphoma or carcinoma of the cecum. If there is a fever or a fistula, diverticulitis may be suspected. Even in established Crohn's, it may not be possible to distinguish a mass due to thickened bowel from that of a complicating abscess.

When diarrhea is predominant, the many other causes of diarrhea must be excluded (see Chapter 8). If colitis is not found on sigmoidoscopy, a small-bowel enema should establish the diagnosis (see the following).

SMALL-BOWEL CROHN'S DISEASE

The principal manifestations of small-bowel Crohn's disease are similar to those of ileocecal disease. The narrowed rigid segments of jejunum produce pain in a similar manner (see Figure 14-2). The mechanism of diarrhea is similar as well, but malabsorption of nutrients and bacterial overgrowth may be more important than the derangement of bile salt metabolism. Because narrowing is higher in the gut, vomiting may be a prominent feature. The principal differences from ileocecal Crohn's are the difficulty in making a diagnosis, and the nutritional consequences.

The small bowel, especially the jejunum, is the least accessible segment of the gut. An endoscopist or radiologist can easily examine the upper gut as far as the mid-duodenum, and the colon to the terminal ileum, but small-bowel examination is more challenging. The disease may be demonstrated by a *small-bowel follow-through* examination. Here barium is swallowed and permitted to trickle through the gut. The loops of bowel often overlap one another, however, and intestinal secretions quickly dilute the barium. The more effective *small-bowel enema* avoids these pitfalls and is quicker to perform (Figures 12-1 and 27-8). Also called *enteroclysis*, this procedure involves injection of barium through a nasogastric tube placed in the duodenum, rapidly filling the intestine with barium. Sadly, however, even this procedure may disappoint the experts. Finally, an enteroscope has been developed to examine the small bowel endoscopically, but it is not yet a practical instrument because of difficulty in passing the instrument, and poor visibility in the narrow, tortuous small-bowel loops.

For these reasons, the diagnosis of small-bowel Crohn's is sometimes delayed. One child of 8 years had no appetite, vomited frequently, and failed to grow. She had no diarrhea and little pain, so small-bowel disease was not considered until the age of 12. In the meantime, she was thought to have anorexia nervosa. A middle-aged woman had infrequent, severe attacks of crampy abdominal pain and vomiting, but between attacks was well. All standard x-rays, including a small-bowel follow-through, were negative, blood work and sedimentation rate were normal, and extensive

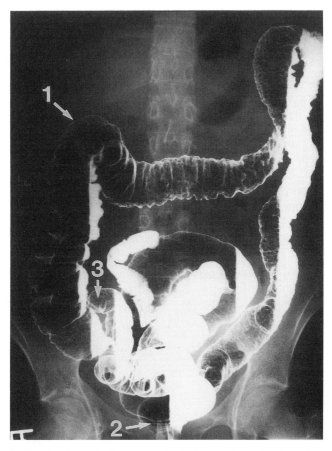

Figure 12-2. Colonic Crohn's disease. This is an air-contrast barium enema showing many tiny white collections of barium studding most regions of the colon. These represent small mucosal ulcers. The normal haustral pattern is absent. Compare to normal barium enema (Figure 27-9). The skip area in the hepatic flexure (1), the rectal sparing (2), and the tiny ulcers in the terminal ileum (3) distinguish Crohn's from ulcerative colitis.

small-bowel Crohn's was detected only after several years by a meticulous small-bowel enema. In an older patient, one may not think of the diagnosis. At least early on, small-bowel disease may be quite indolent. Strictures and even fistulas may develop subtly with few signs of inflammation.

The jejunum is the principal site of absorption of most nutrients, excepting only iron and vitamin B_{12}, which are absorbed in the duodenum and ileum, respectively. This long segment has the greatest absorbing surface because of deep folds and long villi, on whose mucosal surfaces are digestive enzymes such as lactase and the peptidases. The products of digestion are released in the jejunal lumen. Not surprisingly, therefore, small-bowel Crohn's produces the most profound nutritional consequences. Although the ileum, as a reserve, may capture nutrients that escape absorption in the jejunum, it may itself be diseased or resected, or nutrients may not reach that far.

Nutrients are malabsorbed in jejunal disease, and protein and other vital substances are lost from its weeping, inflamed surface. Further, the patient may suffer sitophobia. (Sitophobia is not fear of seeing, but rather fear of eating because of subsequent pain and vomiting.)

A stricture may permit bacteria to grow in the normally sterile small bowel. These may destroy bile salts necessary for fat digestion, or consume vitamin B_{12} before it can be absorbed. The nutritional consequences of Crohn's disease are discussed in Chapters 14 and 25. Suffice it to say here that they are most profound in small-bowel disease, and are of special significance during the growth and development of children.

COLONIC CROHN'S
(GRANULOMATOUS COLITIS)

Unlike those of small-bowel or ileocecal disease, the clinical manifestations of colonic Crohn's more closely resemble those of ulcerative colitis. In fact, if the left colon is involved, both physician and pathologist sometimes may be unable to distinguish the two.

Whereas small bowel disease has obstructive and nutritional consequences, colitis causes crampy diarrhea, urgency, and often bleeding. Although colonic strictures do occur, they are less likely to obstruct.

There are significant differences from ulcerative colitis (see Table 11-1). The rectum is often spared, and there may be more than one involved segment in the colon and small bowel (Figure 12-2). In the early stages of Crohn's before deep ulcers occur, the diarrhea may be less bloody than that found in ulcerative colitis. Unlike the carpet of microulcers seen in the latter disease, the mucosa in Crohn's often appears swollen and thickened, and the ulcers are larger, deeper, and arranged along the long axis of the colon. Later a swollen mucosa among deep ulcers produces a pavement or cobblestone appearance. In advanced ulcerative colitis, on the other hand, mucosal islands stand out as pseudopolyps against the denuded mucosa (see Figure 7-2).

Anal disease, fistulas, and abscesses are more a feature of Crohn's than of ulcerative colitis. Because inflammation involves all layers in the former, an abdominal mass and local tenderness are more likely. When disease is confined to the right colon, it is more likely to be Crohn's. Those infectious agents that may first be mistaken for ulcerative colitis may also be mistaken for Crohn's (Chapter 8). In particular, yersinia, campylobacter, and, in some countries, tuberculosis may produce a right-sided colitis that initially resembles Crohn's disease.

PERIANAL CROHN'S DISEASE

Disease of the perineum is the most emotionally devastating variety of Crohn's disease. The deep, painful, disfiguring anal fistulas can be debilitating and destroy sexual relationships. Usually other segments of the gut are involved, and facilitate the recognition of perianal Crohn's. When the disease begins with an anal fissure or fistula, however, the cause may be less evident. The wary surgeon will not operate on anal disease without first examining the bowel, because healing and repair of tissues affected by Crohn's disease is notoriously poor. Nevertheless, skilled surgery is often required eventually, especially if an abscess develops.

An anal fissure is a tear in the anal mucosa. Simple fissures often result from the traumatic passage of hard, constipated stools, frequent liquid stools, or overzealous wiping. Passage of stool over the fissured area can be exquisitely painful. Softening or bulking the stool with bran or psyllium, and gentle cleansing techniques, usually suffice to heal a fissure. Occasionally, in chronic fissures, the surgeon is forced to excise the lesion, or reduce spasm by partially cutting the anal sphincter. The diseased anal tissues of perianal Crohn's do not permit quick success with these measures, and the surgeon's hand is stayed until every alternative approach has been exhausted.

The anal crypts where colon mucosa merges with perianal skin are often the initial sites of inflammation. A fistula may track inward to form an abscess behind the sphincter. From here fistulas may track in virtually every direction. They may penetrate the wall to surface in the perianal skin, vagina, bladder, or a more proximal segment of the gut. If no outlet is reached, white cells and bacteria gather in the damaged and dying tissue to form an abscess. In the skin surrounding the anus, a fistula may appear as a tiny sinus draining pus or feces. The sinus may connect with the gut through the anal sphincter, or any point above, and may be very difficult to treat.

OTHER

Any segment of the gut may be involved with Crohn's disease, but disease above the jejunum is uncommon, except for that in the mouth. Mouth lesions are white, superficial, painful ulcers. They are similar to the aphthous ulcers or cankers occasionally experienced by most people. In Crohn's, however, the ulcers are multiple, persistent, involve the whole oral cavity and throat, and tend to occur with attacks of Crohn's elsewhere in the gut.

The esophagus is so rarely involved, the diagnosis may not even be considered. In an older person, one may think of reflux esophagitis, which often complicates prednisone therapy. Debilitated patients, or those on steroids or immunosuppressive drugs, may get a monilial (fungal) infection of the esophagus. Gastric Crohn's is also rare, and is discovered accidently or in conjunction with disease elsewhere. The first sign of duodenal Crohn's is often bleeding. A barium x-ray or endoscopy demonstrates a deformed duodenum, leading to confusion with the much commoner duodenal ulcer.

Although we choose to group Crohn's disease into several varieties according to the segment of gut involved, combinations may occur. Perianal Crohn's may accompany ileocecal Crohn's. In an obscure colitis, the discovery of small-bowel disease may clinch the diagnosis of Crohn's disease. In ileocecal disease there may be another involved segment higher up. Upper gastrointestinal tract Crohn's is seldom an isolated phenomenon. Because the segment involved determines the clinical manifestations, their interpretation should indicate the choice of examination.

DIAGNOSIS

In western countries, a young person who presents with a several-week history of increasing diarrhea, fever, cramps, and a tender abdominal mass above the right groin poses little diagnostic challenge. The white blood cell count, platelets, and sedimentation rate are generally elevated. Frequently the patient is treated for ileocecal Crohn's on the basis of this clinical evidence. More detailed information about the extent and location of the disease may be sought later. A principal concern is to distinguish an ileocecal mass due to Crohn's from an abscess. Ultrasound examination is a noninvasive test that may confirm the thickened small-bowel loops of regional enteritis, and help exclude an abscess due to a Crohn's fistula, or a perforated appendix. A sigmoidoscopy, although it does not permit examination of the ileocecal area, may disclose the aphthous ulcers of early Crohn's or even a frank colitis. The physician may take the opportunity at sigmoidoscopy to inspect the perineum for signs of perianal Crohn's disease (see Chapter 27).

Difficulties may arise when the onset is acute and appendicitis is considered, or in the elderly, in whom diverticulitis or a malignant cause is more likely. In the Third World, intestinal tuberculosis is common. Ultrasound may help here as well. If no mass is observed, infectious diarrhea might explain the symptoms, so stool cultures should be obtained.

When the disease is suspected to be in the small intestine, a small-bowel enema as described previously is the investigative technique likely to provide the most information on the nature, extent, and location of the disease (see Figure 27-8). Some might attempt a colonoscopy, but for several reasons I think this is unwise. It is an expensive, painful test. In a young person with a new chronic disorder, colonoscopy may be frightening and impair the doctor–patient rapport, which is so essential to successful management. Even in good hands, the colonoscope may not reach the cecum. In any case, the involvement of the small bowel is of more import than that of right colon, so that in ileocecal disease, detailed examination of the right colon adds little useful information. If fistulas are suspected, they are best demonstrated by a barium enema. Computerized tomography (CT) is indicated only if an abscess is suspected after ultrasound, or if the diagnosis remains obscure after a small-bowel enema. As mentioned earlier, the diagnosis is sometimes much delayed. If the history is suggestive of small-bowel disease, and there are systemic signs of inflammation such as fever, anemia, or increased white cell count, it might be justified to repeat the tests after an interval.

When the left colon is involved, one must distinguish Crohn's from ulcerative colitis, or the many infectious causes. The latter have been dealt with in Chapter 8. In the colon, scattered tiny aphthous ulcers, similar to those seen in the mouth, are the earliest lesions of Crohn's disease. Sigmoidoscopic biopsy may show a granuloma close to the ulcer to help support a diagnosis of Crohn's or granulomatous colitis (see Figure 11-3). Crohn's colitis should be suspected, as distinct from ulcerative colitis, when there are large, irregular ulcers separated by relatively unaffected mucosa. In advanced disease, the submucosal swelling and deep ulcers produce the characteristic cobblestone effect. Fistulas, stricture, perianal disease, or an abdominal mass favor Crohn's. Despite these differences, it may be impossible to distinguish the two diseases for many years. Initially, prednisone and the 5-aminosalicylic acid (5-ASA) compounds are effective treatment for both diseases. Distinction becomes more important later when one contemplates the use of drugs specific for Crohn's, such as metronidazole, or 6-mercaptopurine (6-MP), or the performance of a curative colectomy for ulcerative colitis.

Severe perianal disease in a young person should suggest Crohn's disease. Benign fissures are tiny, almost impossible to see, like a paper cut. Passage of stool over such a lesion produces a searing anal pain disproportionate to its size. In Crohn's perianal disease, the surrounding tissues are inflamed and thickened, but the pain is no less intense. One young man with such a lesion termed defecation "a religious experience." Anal fistulas or abscesses seldom occur spontaneously, and should always warn of Crohn's. The small bowel may be affected in persons with perianal Crohn's, so a small-bowel enema is an important diagnostic test. Diagnosis is also facilitated by recognition of concurrent extraintestinal complications of inflammatory bowel disease, such as iritis, erythema nodosum, or rheumatoid spondylitis (Chapter 16).

SUMMARY

Any segment of the gut may be affected in Crohn's disease. The common varieties are ileocecal, small-bowel, colonic, and perianal Crohn's disease. Rarely the upper gut may be involved. Skip areas are common, and two or more varieties of Crohn's may coexist. Crampy abdominal pain occurs in most varieties, because the normal gut above the lesion must contract vigorously to propel contents through the dysfunctioning and often narrow segment. The transmural nature of the disease produces local pain, mass, and tenderness when the disease is active. Small-intestinal disease causes diarrhea through the malabsorption of nutrients or bile salts; exudation of fluid, protein, and salts from the inflamed surface; bacterial overgrowth; and increased peristalsis. In colonic Crohn's, the mechanisms of diarrhea are similar to those of ulcerative colitis

(Chapter 8). Bleeding may be occult, and is usually less than that in ulcerative colitis. Rarely there may be a massive hemorrhage. As in ulcerative colitis, the chronic inflammation results in fever, weight loss, malaise, malnutrition, and anemia. In small-bowel disease, these manifestations are compounded by malabsorption. The diagnosis of small-bowel Crohn's is often, of necessity, made on clinical grounds, but a small-bowel enema is usually required later for confirmation. A sigmoidoscopy is useful to demonstrate perianal disease, discover early colitis, and confirm most cases of Crohn's colitis. A barium enema is occasionally required to observe the right colon or diagnose enteric fistula, whereas colonoscopy is over-employed and seldom crucially indicated.

CHAPTER THIRTEEN

Crohn's Disease
Treatment

Despite its many similarities to ulcerative colitis, Crohn's disease has several distinctions that compel differences in management. In ulcerative colitis, the extent and severity of the disease determine the graded therapeutic response. Although these parameters are important in Crohn's disease, treatment must also be tailored to the region of the gut that is affected. Further, whereas total colectomy offers an ultimate cure for ulcerative colitis, no such option exists for Crohn's, for which surgery is only palliative. The absence of a cure and frequent steroid dependence have provoked the employment of toxic drugs not ordinarily recommended for the treatment of ulcerative colitis; also, the complications of Crohn's disease discussed in the next chapter are different from those of ulcerative colitis. Nevertheless, the treatments of these two conditions have many similarities, especially when only the colon is involved. The following is a discussion of the management of ileocecal, small-bowel, colitic, perianal, and recurrent Crohn's disease. Ileocecal disease is the prototype against which the others are compared. Detailed discussions of the drugs, diet, and surgery employed in the treatment of Crohn's disease appear in Part 5 of this book.

ILEOCECAL CROHN'S DISEASE

Diagnosis of this most common variant of Crohn's disease is described in Chapter 11. Symptoms result from the acute and chronic inflammation of the gut wall, and the impairment of passage of intestinal contents through the ileocecal lumen. The former causes local abdominal pain, tenderness, swelling, and diarrhea, as well as the systemic features of anemia, fever, and malaise. The latter produces crampy small-bowel contractions, vomiting, and sometimes complete obstruction. To the extent that the obstruction is due to inflammation as opposed to permanent scar, medical management can be expected to improve these manifestations. As with ulcerative colitis, ileocecal Crohn's periodically occurs in attacks, with intervening periods of quiescence. The strategy of management is to treat each attack promptly and with vigor, and withdraw medication at the earliest opportunity. Until recently there has been little proof that any medication prevents recurrent attacks. Often a maintenance dose is required for a time to suppress continuing disease activity. Throughout, one must be wary of the complications of abscess, fistula, perforation, or massive hemorrhage, the treatments of which are discussed in the next chapter. Septic complications require special vigilance, because they may be masked by the anti-inflammatory effect of steroids.

Rest and good nutrition are necessary to maximize the recovery. Ambulatory patients may feel better with a fluid, then soft diet, while waiting for the drugs to act. Dietary supplements such as Ensure may provide calories that are difficult to acquire otherwise. There is an association between smoking and Crohn's disease. Whether this is a causative relationship or not is unknown, but the practice should be stopped anyway.

For attacks of ileocecal Crohn's disease, prednisone is the drug of choice. The principles of its use are similar to those described for ulcerative colitis in Chapter 9. If the attack is moderate, and ambulatory care is possible, oral prednisone is prescribed in a dose of 40 milligrams (eight 5-milligram tablets) per day, usually in divided doses. Improvement may take days or weeks but, once achieved, the dose must be reduced in weekly steps (e.g., 40, 30, 25,

20, 17.5, 15, 12.5, 10, 7.5, 5, 2.5, 0 milligrams per day). Should the disease return, or improvement stall, the dose of the previous week is restored, and maintained for a period. The objective is to reduce the dose to zero as soon as possible, so the undesirable effects of the steroid are minimized. This often implies repeated attempts to reduce the dose below maintenance levels. Despite the efficacy of this treatment, patients may be discouraged by their inability to part with the drug, or the promptness with which the disease recurs following its cessation. Nevertheless, in deference to those unwanted effects of steroids discussed in Chapter 22, the principle of minimal effective therapy should prevail.

Sometimes, a patient undergoing an attack of ileocecal disease is too ill to be treated outside the hospital. Timely admission is essential if control of the disease is to be obtained before complications or malnutrition intervenes. Initially nothing is given by mouth, and fluids, minerals, and vitamins are replenished through an intravenous line. Steroids are given through the same line, and a usual dose is 20 milligrams of methylprednisolone sodium succinate (Solu-Medrol) every 8 or 12 hours.

Pain relief may be afforded by acetaminophen (Tylenol), or meperidine hydrochloride (Demerol) if necessary. Opiate drugs, other than Demerol, such as codeine or morphine, are best avoided for pain or diarrhea control. They are addicting, and their constipating effect may complicate an impending obstruction.

Remission may take 2 or 3 weeks, so nutrition must soon be attended to. If the obstructive symptoms are minimal, clear fluids, and then a light, low-residue diet may be started over a few days. Liquid supplements or an elemental diet may be considered (see Chapter 25). In severe cases in which malnutrition exists, or surgery is not an immediate option, total parenteral (intravenous) nutrition (TPN) may be required. Once feeding has been reestablished, and a remission achieved, the patient may be discharged with step-wise reductions in the steroids.

In the event that obstructive symptoms do not improve, or that high-dose steroids are required over several months, one must consider a surgical "respite," an appropriate term, because recurrence is inevitable. However, a timely resection of the ileocecum, or local relief of an obstinate stricture may have a dramatic, if temporary, beneficial effect. The resulting complete remission of the disease permits tapering of the steroids and normal nutrition. The remission may last many years. Although relapses are similar to the original disease, they may be milder. Nonetheless, the decision to operate must be carefully weighed. Loss of small gut may impair absorption, particularly if the disease recurs in that area, and further surgery becomes necessary. These matters are further discussed in Chapter 26.

The foregoing describes the standard treatment of ileocecal Crohn's disease. Other options, which include diet therapy, newer 5-aminosalicylic acid (5-ASA) compounds, newer steroids, and immunosuppressive drugs, are discussed subsequently.

SMALL-BOWEL CROHN'S DISEASE

The foremost distinction between small-bowel and ileocecal Crohn's is that the jejunum is the least expendable segment of the gut; thus, nutritional considerations assume great importance. The use of steroids and other measures are similar to those described for ileocecal Crohn's, but surgical resection should be avoided wherever possible. Even when necessary, surgery should confine itself to the relief of complications, such as stricture, rather than attempted extirpation of the disease. An earlier belief that all the disease should be removed resulted in "short bowels," condemning their owners to chronic malnutrition and even lifetime TPN.

The adolescent with small-bowel Crohn's disease has special problems. All means, including nutritional manipulation, TPN, even preemptive minimal surgery, may be required to ensure maturation before the bony growth plates fuse (see Chapters 25 and 26).

CROHN'S COLITIS

Disease confined to the right, or proximal, colon may be treated in a manner similar to that for ileocecal disease and will not be further mentioned here. More commonly the left or entire colon is involved. Initially at least, the treatment is similar to that for ulcerative colitis. This is discussed in Chapter 9, and I will emphasize the differences in this section. As in ulcerative colitis, the 5-ASA compounds, especially sulfasalazine, mesalamine (Asacol), and olsalazine (Dipentum) are useful in treatment of mild or moderate disease. Steroids are the treatment of choice in severe disease. Topical therapy with these drugs may be employed if the rectum is involved. Although it is useful in ulcerative colitis, sulfasalazine has not been proven prophylactic when given between attacks, so that the medication is generally stopped when remission is achieved. It does appear, though, that mesalamine (Asacol) in a dose of 800 milligrams three times a day for 1 year is effective in maintaining remission, even in ileal disease.

Unlike ulcerative colitis, Crohn's disease may affect other segments of the gut, and is especially prone to perianal complications. These may modify the management plan. Surgery cannot offer a cure for Crohn's disease, so total colectomy is a last resort. Even though the colon is relatively expendable, the possibility of recurrence haunts the Crohn's patient; therefore, an ileal pouch–anal anastomosis is not an option (see Chapter 26).

In Crohn's disease of the colon, metronidazole appears to be as effective as sulfasalazine. It therefore is an option where steroids or 5-ASA have failed. Perhaps because of its antimicrobial action, it seems to offer particular advantages where fistulas or septic complications exist. The usual dose is 250 milligrams three or four times a day. Metallic taste, low white cell count, peripheral nerve damage, and other side-effects are discussed in Chapter 23.

PERIANAL CROHN'S DISEASE

Perianal Crohn's is the most vexing of all the variants. As discussed in Chapter 11, healing of perianal lesions is very poor, and surgery is fraught with complications. Local surgery should be reserved for situations in which a large, painful abscess threatens general sepsis or local destruction of the anal sphincter. In such a situation, the surgeon will attempt to drain the abscess and excise the fistula. In extreme cases a temporary colostomy may be necessary to divert the fecal stream and permit healing. Unfortunately, such a colostomy may become permanent.

Because of the unsatisfactory results of surgery, vigorous medical treatment should be pursued. Steroids and 5-ASA seem to have little effect; indeed, steroids may be counterproductive in the face of an abscess. Metronidazole may be helpful. Through its antibiotic effect, it destroys the anaerobic bacteria that reside in the abscess. Perhaps through this and other effects it permits healing of the fistula. There are many anecdotes describing healing of fistulas with azathioprine or 6-mercaptopurine (6-MP). These are toxic drugs, and the fistulas appear to recur once treatment is withdrawn. Clearly more effective therapy is needed.

More than any other form of inflammatory bowel disease (IBD), perianal Crohn's requires attention to the victim's psychosocial state. No other manifestation so threatens, or appears to threaten, the patient's future happiness. There is usually sex, marriage, and children in such a patient's future, but much patience, reassurance, and understanding are required to help the often very young patient through the active phases of the disease (see Chapter 19).

RECURRENT CROHN'S DISEASE

Recurrence of disease following resection of an affected segment of bowel is to be expected. This may occur almost right away, or after an interval of as many as 20 years or more. Most often, the disease recurs just proximal to the anastomosis, that is, where the two gut ends are joined by the surgeon (see Figure 26-4). In most cases there is some colonoscopic evidence of recurrence within three months of the surgery. Recurrences are often clinically similar to the original disease; that is, if the surgery was for obstruction, the recurrence tends to feature obstruction, and so on with abscesses, fistulas, and symptoms. Disease may also recur in an ileostomy. If there are significant symptoms, treatment is usually similar to that described for ileocecal disease.

After large or multiple resections, nutrition may be threatened by further surgery, which limits the treatment options; therefore, the operation is delayed as long as possible. Even then, a minimal procedure, such as stricturoplasty for obstruction, is preferred.

ALTERNATIVE TREATMENTS

Dietary Therapy

Certainly good nutrition is an essential ingredient in management of Crohn's disease, especially of the small bowel. Beyond this, there is enthusiasm on the part of some for the use of diet as treatment. I mention, only to condemn, the myriad quack diets touted by self-styled diet therapists to a vulnerable clientele. There are, however, three approaches that are the subject of legitimate study. They are parenteral nutrition, elimination diet, and elemental diet. The brief discourse here is supplemented by a more complete discussion in Chapter 25.

If a luminal factor is thought to be the trigger for the inflammatory response, why not attempt to eliminate it? All three approaches described here might accomplish this. Absolute elimination of a luminal factor is accomplished through TPN. Here all the essential nutrients, calories, vitamins, and minerals are delivered through an intravenous device inserted into a large neck vein (see Figure 25-2). Although an important method of nourishing the patient with malnutrition or multiple surgeries, TPN, by itself, does not appear to possess healing power in Crohn's disease.

Workers in Cambridge, England, have evolved an elaborate elimination diet whereby potential inciting factors, such as wheat, eggs, or beef, are excluded from the diet. When remission is complete, these are systematically and blindly reintroduced, one at a time. This cumbersome procedure is not widely adopted, and its success is doubtful.

In an elemental diet, simple sugars, fats, and amino acids that provide energy and building materials for protein are included, along with essential vitamins and minerals. These are the normal end-products of digestion and may be too small to incite an immune response. If total removal of foreign substances from the gut through TPN is ineffective, why should one believe an elemental diet will help induce a remission? The answer is that an unfed gut may atrophy from disuse and malnourishment. A fed gut is a more healthy gut. Nevertheless, despite some encouraging work from Dublin and the United Kingdom, these diets are rarely employed on their own in North America. Each available commercial product (Flexical, Vivonex, Vital, and Tolerex) has its own special virtue; however, they have in common great expense and deplorable taste, which limit their practicality. Sometimes, they must be administered through a nasogastric tube. Few physicians employ these diets alone in the treatment of an exacerbation of Crohn's disease, but some recommend them along with steroids in a severe attack. There is as yet little evidence that such an approach is justified, and apart from providing nourishment, elemental diets may not justify their expense in the treatment of Crohn's disease (see Chapter 25).

New 5-ASA Preparations

Recently, several new 5-ASA products (see Chapter 20) have been introduced, which employ novel methods of delivering 5-ASA to the colon and which, unlike sulfasalazine, do not contain sulfonamide. Two of these, Salofalk and Pentasa (mesalamine) release 5-ASA in the small intestine and are proposed for the treatment of ileocecal and small-bowel Crohn's disease, respectively. There are anecdotal reports of success, but controlled trials are lacking. They may be worthy of consideration in the steroid-dependent patient with small-bowel disease.

New Steroids

Budesonide is a new steroid (see Chapter 21) absorbed in the small bowel, but destroyed in its first pass via the portal vein through the liver. Thus the drug is delivered intact to the area of therapeutic need, but does not survive in the bloodstream long enough to exert the undesirable systemic effects of steroids. Budesonide or a similar steroid promises to revolutionize the treatment of IBD, but studies are at an early stage.

Immunosuppressives

Azathioprine and 6-MP are the two immunosuppressives with which we have accumulated the most experience in the treatment of Crohn's disease. Because 6-MP is a metabolic product of azathioprine, the two drugs are often considered the same. A large, multicentered United States trial reported in 1979 that azathioprine was ineffective by itself, but that it permitted use of a lower dose of steroid. There are design faults in this trial, which critics say explain the failure to demonstrate benefit. For example, they say the dose was small and fixed, and the duration of treatment, too short. In 1980 a small study showed that 6-MP affords benefit to Crohn's disease not achieved by placebo. Favorable reports of many uncontrolled studies have appeared since. For more details, refer to Chapter 22.

Despite a lack of satisfying proof, there seems little doubt that these drugs produce some benefit for some sufferers of Crohn's disease, but there are other factors of concern. Azathioprine and 6-MP appear to require administration for 3 months before any benefit is realized, so they are of little use in severe exacerbations. Once started, they are not easy to withdraw and seem to be required for many years. Pancreatitis and bone marrow depression are serious, if rare, side-effects. Immunosuppressives may have some long-term genetic consequences and, some believe, may permit cancers to develop. Therefore, the decision to use these drugs cannot be undertaken lightly. They are contraindicated in pregnancy and are best avoided in the very young. The patient must be aware of the side-effects, and regular monitoring of the white blood count is essential. Despite these caveats, for the steroid-resistant or steroid-dependent patient with Crohn's disease in whom surgery is not an option, 6-MP may provide welcome respite.

The search for less toxic, more effective immunosuppressives has motivated trials of cyclosporine and methotrexate. Despite early favorable reports, we must await the results of ongoing clinical trials of these potentially dangerous drugs in Crohn's disease before introducing them into clinical practice.

SUMMARY

As with ulcerative colitis, the extent and severity of the disease are major determinants of the therapeutic attack. In Crohn's disease, however, the segment of gut affected assumes great importance as well. Unlike ulcerative colitis, Crohn's disease cannot be cured, so long-term steroids or toxic immunosuppressives are often forced on the patient by the disease. Prednisone is the cornerstone of drug management, and the 5-ASA drugs are effective in colonic disease. Some of the new 5-ASA drugs are released in the small gut and may prove effective there. Immunosuppressives should be reserved for patients with previous surgeries who are steroid dependent or steroid resistant. Treatment should be graded to reflect the severity of the attack. More severe cases may require hospitalization for intravenous steroids, nutritional support, and symptom control. Although the importance of special diets to nutrition is obvious, diet as treatment of Crohn's disease is controversial. Elemental diet especially deserves more study. Crohn's disease tends to go into remission, and attacks may be infrequent. One should take advantage of a remission to withdraw the steroids in steps and shore up nutrition. Occasionally continuously active disease requires maintenance steroids at the lowest effective dose for a time. On the basis of current information, prophylaxis with large-dose 5-ASA during remission appears to be effective.

CHAPTER FOURTEEN

Crohn's Disease
Complications

Because of the distinct pathology of Crohn's disease, its complications are different from those of ulcerative colitis (Table 14-1). Recall first that all three layers of the gut are involved in the inflammatory process. As a result, mucosal ulcers may extend through the gut wall and beyond to produce fistula, abscess, or even free perforation into the peritoneal cavity. The deep ulcers may bleed, producing blood loss and iron-deficiency anemia. Recall also that any level of the gut may be involved. Fulminant colitis, toxic megacolon, and even colon cancer do occur in Crohn's colitis, albeit much less frequently than in ulcerative colitis, but when Crohn's disease involves the small intestine, unique complications result. The narrow small-gut lumen is susceptible to obstruction. Disease of the ileum impairs the absorption of vitamin B_{12} and bile salts, whereas disease in the jejunum may cause severe malabsorption and growth retardation.

TABLE 14-1
Complications of Crohn's Disease

Life-threatening
  Obstruction
  Fistula
  Abscess
  Perforation
  Massive hemorrhage
  Toxic megacolon
  Colon cancer
Non-life-threatening
  Anemia
  Malnutrition
  Growth retardation

LIFE-THREATENING COMPLICATIONS

Obstruction

In small-bowel and ileocecal Crohn's disease, the thickened, inflamed bowel narrows the lumen. When this narrowing reaches a critical point where the passage of intestinal contents is halted, small-bowel obstruction (Figure 14-1) is said to have occurred. The obstruction may be complete or incomplete (subacute). The small-intestinal muscle above the obstruction contracts vigorously, and the patient experiences painful cramps. When the obstruction is high in the intestine, food is backed up, and vomiting occurs. Air and fluid, moved by gut contractions, gurgle and splash. These exaggerated bowel sounds may be heard by the patient or detected by the physician through a stethoscope. The abdomen becomes distended and tender, especially if there is actively inflamed bowel. Abdominal plain x-rays show dilated loops of small bowel with air–fluid levels, and if the obstruction is complete, there is no air in the colon (Figure 14-1).

There are two components to the obstruction of Crohn's disease. The first is the inflammation and swelling of active disease.

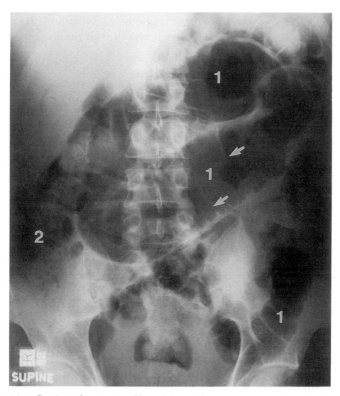

Figure 14-1. Supine plain x-ray film of the abdomen showing incomplete small-bowel obstruction due to Crohn's disease of the ileum. Note the dilated loops of small bowel (1). The circular folds around the lumen (arrows) distinguish small bowel from the haustral pattern of the colon. See Figure 27-6 for comparison. The presence of air (and feces) in the ascending colon (2) indicates that the obstruction is incomplete.

This component is usually reversible with time and treatment. The other component is scarring, which is not reversible. Scarring usually results after repeated attacks of active Crohn's, but may occasionally be the first manifestation of a chronic, subclinical process. Which of these two components is dominant determines whether an obstructive episode will respond to medical treatment, or require surgical intervention.

An obstructive episode in Crohn's is managed with intravenous fluids and salts to provide daily needs and compensate for fluid losses into the dilated gut. Naturally nothing should be taken by mouth, and if vomiting occurs, a tube is passed through the nose and throat into the stomach to decompress the gut. Continuous suction is often applied to the tube. Intravenous steroids [methylprednisolone (Solu-Medrol) 20 milligrams every 8 or 12 hours] reduces the inflammation. To the extent that this is successful, the patient should soon have the nasogastric tube removed, and begin feeding, first with fluids, later with a soft diet. If the narrowed bowel is due to fibrous strictures, the obstruction will not regress, and surgery becomes inevitable. As discussed in Chapter 26, extensive resection is best avoided. Usually the surgeon will do minimal surgery, sometimes a refashioning of the stricture to widen the lumen (stricturoplasty). Often there are several strictures (Figure 14-2).

Fistula

When deep ulcers become channels through the gut wall, they are called fistulas (Figure 14-3). They may track to any adjacent organ. Thus there are fistulas to skin (enterocutaneous), bladder (enterovesicle), vagina (enterovaginal), intestine (enterocolic, enteroenteral), and perianal. An enterocutaneous fistula sometimes follows surgery and communicates between gut and skin through the wound. It is often difficult to find the origin of a fistula. Sometimes a sinogram is employed, in which contrast medium is injected into the fistula or sinus where it may be seen by x-ray. Metronidazole and

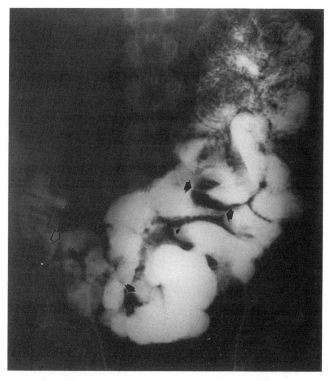

Figure 14-2. Antegrade small-bowel enema demonstrating multiple small-bowel strictures (black arrows). A normal, feathery small-bowel pattern is seen above, and an ileocecal anastomosis (hollow arrow) is the result of a previous ileal resection.

6-mercaptopurine (6-MP) seem to aid fistula healing. Surgery is difficult, but may eventually become necessary.

An enterovesicle fistula is suspected when a person with Crohn's disease has frequent urinary tract infections. It is the most likely explanation for pneumaturia (air in the urine). Enterovaginal fistulas are particularly troublesome and can be psychosocially

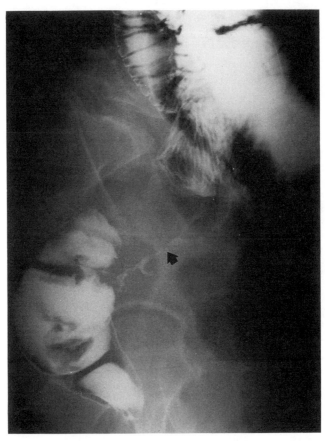

Figure 14-3. Enterosigmoid fistula. This is an antegrade small-bowel enema showing barium from the upper small intestine tracking through a long, narrow fistula (arrow) to the sigmoid colon, so that the rectosigmoid fills with barium, and the remainder of the colon and ileum remain empty. Because so much small bowel is bypassed, and bacteria now contaminate the upper gut, this patient suffered severe malabsorption. Many sinuses may be seen originating from this one long fistula. This fistula might also be detected by barium enema (see text).

devastating. These complications sometimes require a temporary colostomy to redirect the fecal flow and permit healing.

Short enteroenteral or enterocolic fistulas may be of little immediate consequence. If, however, a large segment of the small bowel is bypassed, or overgrown with colon bacteria, malabsorption and weight loss may occur. Diagnosis of such a fistula is not easy, and the colon end is seldom identified by colonoscopy. A barium enema is most likely to demonstrate an enterocolic fistula, whereas a small-bowel enema is most useful for an enteroenteric fistula (Figure 14-3).

A fistula may also occur in colonic diverticulosis, where the infected, perforated diverticulum tracks into a neighboring organ. Rarely a large-bowel cancer may fistulize as well. These considerations apply to older patients and seldom pose a diagnostic problem in the young. In the Third World enteric tuberculosis or the fungus disease actinomycosis may cause fistulas, but in western countries, Crohn's disease is by far the most likely cause.

Abscess

When a fistula tracks into the peritoneal cavity, the resulting infection may be confined to an area within the cavity by mesentery, loops of bowel, and inflammatory tissue to form an abscess (Figure 14-4). Alternatively, an abscess may occur in the pelvic tissues or the perineum, often as a result of the failure to drain of a fistula communicating with the skin or other organ. Such an abscess is a serious illness with high fever, chills, malaise, and even toxicity. The white blood cell count may be high. Usually inhabited by enteric, often anaerobic (no oxygen requirement) organisms, an abscess may infect the blood (septicemia). Sometimes a Crohn's abscess is difficult to recognize, its symptoms masked by those of the enteritis itself, and the antiinflammatory effects of prednisone. Abdominal or pelvic ultrasound, or sometimes computerized tomography (CT scan) will localize the pus collection, which may then be drained through a needle directed by the imaging technique (Figures 14-4 and 14-5). Drainage of the pus is important, and an operation may be

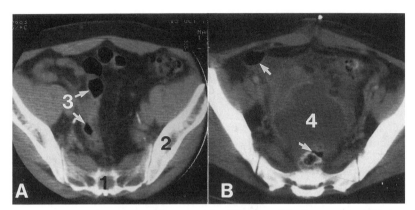

Figure 14-4. (A) Computerized tomography (CT) scan of the lower pelvis. This is a cross-sectional slice seen from below. Note the spine (1), ileac bones of the pelvis (2), and rectosigmoid colon (3). (B) CT scan of a slice similar to that of (A) in a patient with a large pelvic abscess (4) due to Crohn's disease. Note that the loops of rectosigmoid colon are pushed aside. Courtesy of Dr. H. Tao.

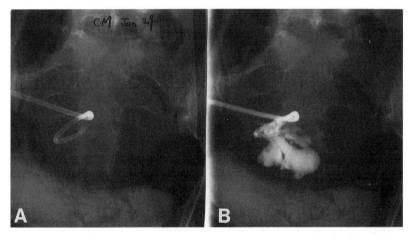

Figure 14-5. (A) Plain film of the pelvis in the patient whose abscess was demonstrated in Figure 14-4 (B). A catheter has been inserted through the abdominal wall into the abscess. (B) Contrast medium has been injected through the catheter into the abscess. The abscess fluid (pus) may be drained through this catheter. Courtesy of Dr. H. Tao.

required. Antibiotic treatment may help prevent spread of the abscess and mop up infection after drainage. It is best, however, if pus can be first obtained and cultured. This permits identification of the offending organism and more accurate selection of antibiotics. If blind therapy is necessary, metronidazole, ampicillin, and gentamycin are typically used in concert to kill most responsible organisms. Imipenem (Primaxin) is an expensive newer antibiotic, which should be reserved for resistant cases.

Free Perforation

Deep, penetrating ulcers may burst through the three layers of the gut into the normally sterile peritoneal space. Fortunately such a catastrophe is rare. The resulting infection is called peritonitis, and is considered a surgical emergency. Under antibiotic cover, the surgeon must quickly move to seal or resect the leak and cleanse the abdominal cavity.

Such a perforation may be announced by the sudden onset of severe abdominal pain. The patient quickly becomes gravely ill, and signs of shock may intervene. The abdomen is silent, rigid, and exquisitely tender. A plain x-ray of the abdomen may clinch the diagnosis through the demonstration of free air (Figure 10-2). The surgeon may be forced to do a temporizing procedure to drain the infection, leaving the repair until the patient is in better shape. Steroids and the immunosuppressant drugs used in the treatment of the underlying Crohn's disease suppress the body's defense mechanisms against infection. This muted response to injury may obscure the signs of perforation; thus, during high-dose steroid treatment, vigilant supervision is important.

Massive Hemorrhage

The ulcers of Crohn's disease ooze blood, and in colitis, blood is often apparent in the stool. Rarely, an ulcer as it burrows through the gut wall may shear an artery and produce a vigorous, life-threatening hemorrhage. Transfusions may be required, along with special measures to optimize blood clotting. Fresh frozen plasma restores clotting factors whose production is impaired by lack of vitamin K. Usually the hemorrhage stops spontaneously, but occasionally an operation is urgently required.

Toxic Megacolon

This complication is much less likely in Crohn's disease than in ulcerative colitis. The precautions and management discussed in Chapter 10 are applicable here.

Colon Cancer

Even in colonic Crohn's disease, the risk of future colon cancer appears to be much less than that in ulcerative colitis. Nevertheless, some experts believe that cancer is more likely in Crohn's than in unaffected people. At this stage of knowledge, colonoscopic surveillance after 10 years of disease, such as that recommended for ulcerative colitis, seems to be unwarranted in Crohn's.

CHRONIC COMPLICATIONS

Anemia

As in ulcerative colitis, anemia may result from chronic blood loss, or bone marrow depression, the so-called *anemia of chronic disease*. Sulfasalazine, commonly used in Crohn's colitis, may introduce a hemolytic anemia, in which healthy red blood cells are destroyed in the spleen and other tissues. In small-bowel disease, failure to ingest or failure to absorb hematinic agents such as iron or folic acid may be important as well.

Iron is plentiful in red meats and is adequate in most diets. Normally a very small amount is needed each day to make up for normal small losses in the intestine, or from menstruation in women. In small-bowel disease, iron losses may outstrip the oral intake or duodenal absorption of iron. An iron-deficient anemia is characterized by small red cells with reduced hemoglobin content (microcytic, hypochromic). Liver stores of folic acid are sufficient for 1 or 2 months, and the vitamin is normally plentiful in the diet. Prolonged failure to ingest or absorb this essential vitamin results in ineffective marrow production of red blood cells. The red cells in this case are large and immature (macrocytic, hyperchromic).

Vitamin B_{12} is absorbed from the ileum. Normal liver stores are usually good for 4 or 5 years, so vitamin B_{12} deficiency is not common in Crohn's disease. Best known as the vitamin that is deficient in pernicious anemia, this third hematinic agent is essential for the maturation of red cells. Long-standing ileal resection may result in an anemia characterized by large, immature cells similar to those seen in folic acid deficiency. In jejunal strictures, overgrowth of B_{12}-consuming organism may, over many years, have a similar result. As in pernicious anemia, this anemia is easily treated and prevented by monthly injections of 100 micrograms of vitamin B_{12}. The bacterial overgrowth may be treated with an antibiotic such as tetracycline.

Malnutrition

Malnutrition (see Chapter 25) may occur in Crohn's disease in a manner similar to that in ulcerative colitis. Intestinal loss of protein, energy consumption by the inflammatory process, tissue breakdown due to steroid therapy, and inadequate diet all contrive to produce weight loss and specific nutritional deficiencies. In small-bowel Crohn's, all this is compounded by failure to absorb nutrients.

When the ileum is involved or resected, bile salts, normally absorbed in this segment of small gut, are lost into the colon, where they have a cathartic effect. This phenomenon may cause a cholerheic diarrhea, depending on how much terminal ileum is lost. The anion-exchange resin cholestyramine (Questran), if taken by mouth, binds the bile salts and prevents their laxative action.

Bile salts are detergents, essential for absorption of fat. Fats are water insoluble, but the electrochemical and detergent effects of bile salts solubilize fats, and encourage their digestion. Bile salts, produced and excreted by the liver, thus arrive in the upper small bowel and permit digestion of fatty acids and cholesterol. The fat-soluble vitamins A, D, E, and K are insoluble in water, and their absorption depends on the presence of bile salts in the gut. In severe ileal disease or resection, therefore, loss of bile salts contributes to weight loss and fat-soluble vitamin deficiencies.

Vitamin K is necessary for the production of certain blood-clotting proteins in the liver. Their deficiency impairs blood clotting and permits bleeding from diseased areas or operative sites. Patients unable to eat or receiving prolonged intravenous therapy may run out of these clotting factors. A test called the prothrombin time (PT) measures the effectiveness of these proteins. The longer the PT, the greater the clotting impairment. Vitamin K deficiency is prevented or treated over a day or two by the intravenous injection of 10 milligrams of vitamin K_1 oxide. Intramuscular injection may cause a local skin reaction. In an emergency, rapid clotting improvement may be achieved by the intravenous administration of fresh frozen plasma, which supplies the missing proteins "ready-made."

Vitamin A deficiency leads to night blindness and skin disease. It is not a common feature of Crohn's disease. Vitamin D deficiency is another matter. The metabolism of vitamin D is very complex and involves the intestine, liver, kidney, and skin. For our purpose, it is important to know that this vitamin is essential for the absorption and regulation of calcium. Calcium and phosphorus combine with protein to form bone. When vitamin D is lacking, the bones become insufficiently calcified. The resulting weak bones bend in children (rickets) or break in adults (osteomalacia). Early osteomalacia may be suspected when the serum calcium and phosphorus are low and the serum alkaline phosphatase is high. The latter is an enzyme that is elevated in some liver disorders, and sophisticated tests may be required to distinguish osteomalacia from other metabolic bone or liver disease. Vitamin D deficiency due to bile salt malabsorption may be aggravated by poor diet and malabsorption of the vitamin and calcium from a diseased jejunum. Vitamin D and calcium supplements are the treatment, but care is necessary not to over-dose. In summer, infrared rays activate vitamin D in the skin, but in winter, supplements are a wise precaution for the patient with small-bowel disease. The demands for vitamin D are greatest in adolescence and pregnancy, mandating supplements in these conditions of life.

Vitamin B_{12} and bile salts are absorbed in the ileum, and iron, in the duodenum, but virtually every other nutrient is assimilated in the jejunum. Impaired protein, fat, and carbohydrate absorption results in muscle and weight loss. Inadequate calcium or magnesium may cause a disorder of neuromuscular transmission called tetany, featuring muscle irritability and spasm of the hands. Deficiencies of the B vitamins and trace metals may occur as well. At least some of these deficiencies should be anticipated in severe Crohn's disease, and may be countered with specific replacement, or in some cases with defined diets. In extreme situations, total parenteral nutrition may be required (Chapter 25).

Growth Retardation

Small-bowel Crohn's disease and the ensuing undernutrition makes growth retardation even more formidable than that found in ulcerative colitis. About one third of affected children experience growth failure, and in some of these, the retardation is permanent. The situation is made more difficult by the natural reluctance of physicians to use immunosuppressives in children. Moreover, unlike that in ulcerative colitis, surgery will not cure the disease and permit future unimpaired growth. Nevertheless, prompt action is necessary if a growth spurt is to be achieved before the bony epiphyses fuse. If the usual medical means fail to improve nutrition and aid growth, a resection of the affected segment may provide the necessary respite. Obviously removal of too much absorbing surface may be counterproductive; however, excision of inflamed tissue, better eating, and relief of obstruction could compensate for loss of some intestinal absorbing surface.

SUMMARY

Because Crohn's disease involves all levels of the gut and all three layers of the gut wall, its complications are more complex and different from those of ulcerative colitis. In colonic disease, the acute complications may be similar to those of colitis; however, the deep ulcers may result in fistula or abscess involving neighboring organs and the perineum (anogenital area). Toxic megacolon and cancer are less likely. Disease in the narrower small bowel causes various degrees of intestinal obstruction. Small-bowel disease, unique to Crohn's, superimposes a variety of nutritional deficiencies that aggravate the anemia, weight loss, and growth retardation that are common in most inflammatory bowel disease. Small-bowel Crohn's disease adds several possible additional consequences of malnourishment, such as osteomalacia, clotting abnormalities, bile salt diarrhea, and malabsorption.

PART FOUR

Topics Related to Inflammatory Bowel Disease

CHAPTER FIFTEEN

Variant Colitis

We don't now the cause of ulcerative colitis and Crohn's disease. We are even uncertain that they are distinct entities; if the disease is confined to the colon, it may be impossible at some stages to distinguish one from the other. Other variant inflammatory bowel diseases (IBDs) of obscure or unknown cause are the subject of this chapter. Seemingly distinct, they have features that suggest a relationship to IBD, or may at least be confused with it. *Microscopic colitis* is a cause of chronic, watery diarrhea, yet on inspection of the colon, nothing is seen. *Collagenous colitis* may be a later stage of this process. Neither seems related to ulcerative colitis, yet they do respond to steroids and 5-aminosalicylic acid (5-ASA). *Diversion colitis* is found when the fecal stream is diverted from a segment of the colon as a result of surgery. *Pouchitis* refers to the inflammation found in the ileoanal pouch created as a rectal substitute following total colectomy for ulcerative colitis or familial polyposis (Chapter 26). Most enigmatic are the *solitary rectal ulcer syndrome* and *colitis cystica profunda*, which may be initially confused with the proctitis of ulcerative colitis or Crohn's disease. The rare Behçet's disease may even more rarely involve the colon. Finally, *factitious colitis* refers to colonic mucosal damage that may result from laxative use or abuse. Although uncommon, these conditions frequently enter into discussions of IBD.

MICROSCOPIC (LYMPHOCYTIC) COLITIS

Chronic, watery diarrhea of unknown cause is one of the most challenging diagnostic problems in gastroenterology. The possibilities are numerous, and the cost of investigation, great. In such a case, there are usually no revealing signs and symptoms, no abnormalities detectable in the blood, and no observed changes on sigmoidoscopy, barium enema, or small-bowel x-ray. Despite this the patient has persistent, watery diarrhea, often with urgency, incontinence, and increased daily stool weight (i.e., > 350 grams/ day).

In a small number of such patients, usually middle-aged women, colon mucosal biopsy will show the features of microscopic or collagenous colitis. In the former, there are lymphocytes within the epithelium, that single layer of cells that lines the colon lumen (Figure 15-1). There may also be epithelial damage, and inflammation beneath, but none of these changes is visible to the naked eye. Because of the unique intraepithelial lymphocytosis, this lesion is sometimes called *lymphocytic colitis.*

Patients with such findings may improve when treated with sulfasalazine [salicylazosulfapyridine (SASP)] or steroids. As a result, some consider microscopic colitis to be a variant of IBD. The findings are distinct, however, and there is no evidence that the former can metamorphose to the latter.

COLLAGENOUS COLITIS

Collagenous colitis is another variant colitis found in middle-aged women with persistent, watery diarrhea. As in microscopic colitis, the sigmoidoscopic appearance of the colon is normal, and the diagnosis may be made only by biopsy. The characteristic histologic feature is a thickening of the collagen layer that lies immediately under the colon epithelium. Collagen is an inert material, produced by fibrous tissue cells (fibrocytes), and is important in the structure of tissues. The layer under the epithelium, called the collagen plate, is normally 2 to 3 microns (millionths of a

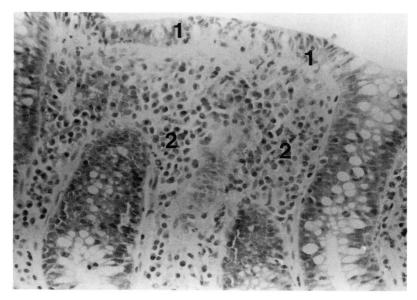

Figure 15-1. Microscopic colitis as seen on colonic mucosal biopsy. Note the lymphocytes invading the epithelium and the damaged epithelial cells (1). There are increased inflammatory cells in the mucosa (2). Photomicrograph courtesy of Dr. M. Guindi. Compare to Figure 1-2.

meter) in thickness. In collagenous colitis, the thickness may be 10 to 60 microns, although the exact upper limit of normal is uncertain (Figure 15-2). This collagen plate is more thickened in the proximal (upper) colon than in the rectum in collagenous colitis, so a proximal biopsy is more likely to confirm the diagnosis. The thickened collagen plate may cause diarrhea by impeding water reabsorption by the colon mucosa.

There is evidence that microscopic and collagenous colitis may be closely related. Both are found predominantly in middle-aged women with watery diarrhea, and both have lymphocytes in the epithelium, with epithelial damage and subepithelial inflammation. In fact, the principal difference, the thickened collagen layer in the latter, has led some to speculate that collagenous colitis is but a later

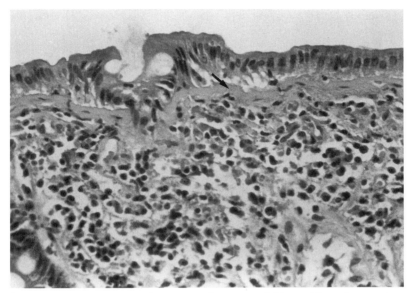

Figure 15-2. Collagenous colitis in a colon mucosal biopsy. The collagen plate under the epithelium is thickened (arrow). Photomicrograph courtesy of Dr. M. Guindi.

stage of microscopic colitis. Such a relationship is further supported by the common improvement in these variants when they are treated with sulfasalazine or steroids. The clinical amelioration is matched by histologic improvement. In contrast, a recent study presents data suggesting that collagenous and microscopic colitis are distinct entities, yet it is the inflammation, not the collagen plate, that causes diarrhea.

The cause of these conditions is unknown. The lymphocytic infiltrate, the predominance in females, and the responses to steroids suggest autoimmunity. The lack of the intestinal, extraintestinal, or systemic features of IBD suggest a mechanism distinct from that of ulcerative colitis or Crohn's disease.

One should conclude that, in a woman with chronic, persistent, watery diarrhea, a colonic epithelial biopsy is indicated, preferably above the rectum. The symptoms of collagenous or microscopic colitis are *not* those of the irritable bowel. The abdominal pain and alternating constipation and diarrhea characteristic of that condition need *not* provoke a colon biopsy.

DIVERSION COLITIS

Several colon diseases may require surgery that results in a colostomy or ileostomy. Occasionally the rectum and distal colon are left in place temporarily so as to minimize surgery in debilitated patients, or permanently, as in the case of colon cancer. The proximal (near) end of the defunctioned segment may be sealed off or sewn to the abdominal wall as a mucous fistula; thus, the fecal stream has been diverted. Normally such an isolated segment of colon discharges a small amount of mucus. Occasionally a colitis develops, producing a troublesome, mucusy, bloody discharge. This diversion colitis may be reversed by reconstituting the colon integrity, and reestablishing the fecal flow.

It is important to distinguish colitis due to diversion from a reactivation of IBD, or a pseudomembranous colitis that might result form the perioperative administration of antibiotics. Sigmoidoscopy, biopsy, and examination of the isolated colon's contents for *Clostridium difficile* should be employed to make this distinction. This colitis seems to result form lack of colon mucosal nutrition by short-chain fatty acids (i.e., butyrate, acetate, propionate), which are normally produced by the colonic bacteria. Local infusion of these short-chain fatty acids appears to improve the colitis. A recent report suggests that the more readily available 5-ASA suppositories may also be effective.

POUCHITIS

Pouchitis is not a colitis at all; rather, it is an inflammation in the ileal pouch—a rectal substitute fashioned by the surgeon after total colectomy for ulcerative colitis or familial polyposis (see Chapter 26). This complication occurs in 10 to 40 percent of ileal pouches. It was previously observed in the continent ileostomy, a pouch opening on the abdominal wall, that is now seldom employed. Pouchitis appears to be more likely if the surgery was done for ulcerative colitis than for familial polyposis.

The clinical features are urgent, watery, often bloody diarrhea with few systemic symptoms. Most cases consist of one or two episodes that respond quickly to a course of metronidazole. The inflammatory changes in the pouch mucosa commence with the establishment of fecal bacteria in the pouch; therefore, anaerobic bacteria such as bacteroides have been blamed for the inflammation. The favorable response to antibiotic therapy in most cases reinforces this view, but the organisms are not eradicated. Inexplicably, the presence or absence of fecal stasis within the pouch seems unimportant.

A smaller number of cases are chronic and resistant to metronidazole. Some of these originally had intermediate colitis as the pathological diagnosis, raising the possibility that this pouchitis is, in fact a recurrence of Crohn's disease. Some with anastomotic inflammation may represent residual colitis in a cuff of colon inadvertently retained by the surgeon. More work is required before we fully understand this entity.

SOLITARY RECTAL ULCER SYNDROME

This enigmatic disease is neither necessarily ulcerating nor solitary. It owes its name to the usual picture of a solitary ulcer on the anterior wall of the rectum, about 7 to 10 centimeters from the anal margin. Sometimes, however, the appearance may be nodular, or similar to that of a proctitis. Only the histologic appearance of a biopsy taken from the affected area confirms the diagnosis. The mucosa is replaced by fibrous tissue, and there is thickening of the narrow muscular layer found under the mucosa (muscularis mucosa).

The cause is thought to be prolapse of rectal mucosa and high intrarectal pressure during defecation. Prolonged straining at stool may traumatize the rectal mucosa, thereby causing ulceration and scarring. Sometimes these phenomena are not obvious. For treatment, the patient may be advised to avoid straining, and to encourage effortless defecation through fiber supplements. Anecdotally, 5-ASA suppositories have been helpful in some cases. There appear to be neither dire consequences, nor cure of this disease, but the alarming appearance may initially raise fears of cancer or IBD.

COLITIS CYSTICA PROFUNDA

Like the solitary rectal ulcer syndrome, this rare condition has been blamed on rectal prolapse; however, it may occur elsewhere in the gut. A modern theory holds that a break in the mucosa becomes a cleft or cyst roofed over by the epithelium. This uncommon condition presents with rectal bleeding, mucus discharge, anal pain, and straining.

The pathology seems distinct. Submucosal cysts may become bulky and fibrotic, leading the examiner on rectal and endoscopic examination to suspect a cancer, or Crohn's disease of the anus. The cysts may be excised, if bleeding or partial obstruction warrant it. The outlook is otherwise benign.

BEHÇET'S DISEASE

This rare disease normally affects the eyes, genitalia, and mouth. There are other features as well, and a few cases of colon involvement have been reported. It may be difficult to differentiate Behçet's disease from a case of IBD in which there are accompanying extraintestinal manifestations, such as iritis and mouth ulcers.

FACTITIOUS COLITIS

Many laxatives, notably bisacodyl (Dulcolax) or phosphate (Fleet) enemas disrupt the colon surface epithelium. In some cases

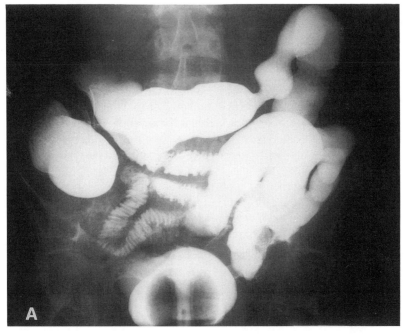

Figure 15-3. Cathartic colon. (A) Barium enema examination of a patient after many years' use of a cascara-containing laxative. The patient had diarrhea, and the lack of haustra in the transverse colon led to the erroneous diagnosis of ulcerative colitis. The colon is elongated, however, not foreshortened, as in ulcerative colitis, and sigmoidoscopy revealed melanosis coli.

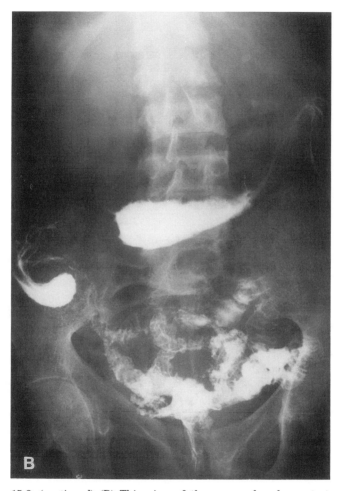

Figure 15-3. (*continued*) (B) This view of the same colon demonstrates long pseudostrictures, another feature of the cathartic colon. Compare to the normal (Figure 27-9) and to the foreshortened colon of chronic ulcerative colitis (Figures 8-2 and 10-5).

there is mild inflammation and goblet (mucous) cell depletion, but normal architecture is restored within 7 days of drug exposure. Mannitol, saline enemas, or per oral colonic lavage (GoLYTELY) cause no such damage. The importance of this histologic phenomenon is its distinction from other forms of colitis.

More profound are the colon changes associated with long-term laxative use and abuse. The chronic use of *stimulant laxatives* such as cascara produces damage to the myenteric nerve plexus in the colon wall. Such a *cathartic colon* is elongated and featureless, without haustra, leading the untrained eye to erroneously interpret a barium enema as chronic ulcerative colitis (Figure 15-3). Long, transient contractions, called pseudostrictures, are characteristic, and there are no ulcers. If the abused laxative is an anthraquinone such as senna or cascara, the colon mucosa may be densely pigmented. Called melanosis coli, this pigmentation disappears within 6 months of cessation of the laxative. Regrettably, the cathartic colon is often irreversible. The principal importance of these observations is that melanosis coli and cathartic colon should not be confused with colitis. They are also evidence of laxative abuse.

OTHER

Nonspecific ulcers may occur rarely in the ascending and transverse colon. Of unknown cause, these may bleed or perforate. A segmental colitis, responsive to 5-ASA and steroids, may occur in an area of diverticula, and is proposed as a variant colitis of the elderly. So-called stercoral ulcers are sometimes found in debilitated patients with severe, long-standing fecal impaction. Therapeutic radiation may induce both acute and chronic colitis. Patients with severe cardiovascular disease have inadequate blood supply to the colon. The result is ischemic colitis. Nonsteroidal antiinflammatory drugs (NSAID) such as ibuprofen (Motrin) or naproxen (Naprosyn) may cause colon ulceration. Ulcers have even been described in the rectums of patients who have deliberately instrumented themselves. These several ulcerating or inflammatory conditions are seldom confused with IBD.

SUMMARY

Distinct from ulcerative colitis or Crohn's disease are several variant colitides. Microscopic and collagenous colitis may be different stages of the same disease process, but the cause of either is unknown. They each cause persistent, watery diarrhea, especially in middle-aged women, yet the radiographic and endoscopic appearances of the colon are normal. Their diagnosis depends on colon mucosal biopsy, and they improve with the administration of sulfasalazine or steroids. A colon segment from which the fecal stream has been diverted may develop a seemingly nutritional colitis. This diversion colitis improves if the fecal flow is restored, or if short-chain fatty acids are locally instilled. Following total colectomy, an ileal pouch is often fashioned as a surrogate rectum. In as many as one third of subjects, pouchitis may occur. Most cases are transient, and respond to metronidazole. Nonresponders raise fears of retained colon mucosa, or an underlying diagnosis of Crohn's disease. Solitary rectal ulcer syndrome is neither solitary, nor necessarily ulcerated. Despite theories, the cause is unknown. Some patients respond to 5-ASA suppositories, and the prognosis seems benign. Colitis cystica profunda is a cystic disorder of the submucosa, which may be related to the solitary rectal ulcer syndrome. Finally, laxatives may acutely damage the colon epithelium, or if used chronically, may result in melanosis coli and the cathartic colon. Other colon mucosal injuries, such as nonspecific ulcers, NSAID ulcers, radiation colitis, or ischemic colitis, are seldom confused with IBD.

CHAPTER SIXTEEN

Extraintestinal Manifestations of IBD

In Chapters 10 and 14 we discussed the complications of ulcerative colitis and Crohn's disease. These occur as direct consequences of the inflamed bowel. Extraintestinal complications are associated diseases in organs other than the intestine whose pathology is distinct from that of inflammatory bowel disease (IBD). Exceptions might be a ureter blocked by an inflammatory Crohn's mass or a Crohn's lesion on the skin. About one fourth of IBD patients have an extraintestinal manifestation. The presence of one increases the likelihood of another. These associations seem more likely in ulcerative colitis or Crohn's disease affecting the colon, than in small-bowel disease. Some of these associated maladies may run a course parallel to that of the IBD, and may even subside with colectomy. Others lead a life of their own. More than 100 of these associations have been described, many of which are probably coincidental. We concentrate on the principal associations, especially those of the joints, skin, liver, eyes, and kidney (Table 16-1). Like that of IBD, the cause of most of these diseases is unknown, but they cast shadows of disordered immunity. Because the focus of this book is IBD, the discussion of these disorders, many of which warrant their own volumes, is necessarily brief.

TABLE 16-1
Extraintestinal Manifestations of IBD

Joint	Ocular
Colitic arthritis	Iritis
Ankylosing spondylitis	Episcleritis
Clubbing	Renal
Skin	Renal complications of Crohn's disease
Erythema nodosum	Kidney stones
Pyoderma gangrenosum	
Aphthous ulcers of the mouth	Pancreatic
Crohn's disease of the skin	Cardiopulmonary
Liver	
Sclerosing cholangitis	Hematologic
Chronic active hepatitis	Thromboembolic
Cirrhosis	Pulmonary embolism
Cholangiocarcinoma	Intravascular clotting and vasculitis
Gallstones	
Other	Amyloidosis

JOINT MANIFESTATIONS

Colitic Arthritis

Colitic arthritis affects the large peripheral joints: knees, hips, ankles, wrists, and elbows, in order of greatest occurrence. Frequently, only one or two joints are involved, and the arthritis may migrate from one to another. The course of the arthritis often parallels that of the IBD, usually of the colon. Blood markers of the common arthritides, such as the rheumatoid factor, are usually absent. A deformed joint may result in some cases. Other extraintestinal diseases are often found with colitic arthritis, particularly erythema nodosum and iritis.

The joint pain, swelling, and stiffness of colitic arthritis follow the course of the colitis, and treatment of the latter may effect great improvement in the former. Patients improve on corticosteroids, and even on sulfasalazine. Colectomy appears to cure the arthritis associated with ulcerative colitis, but the postsurgical outlook is less certain with Crohn's disease.

Ankylosing Spondylitis

Unlike colitic arthritis, ankylosing spondylitis does not follow the course of the associated IBD, nor is it improved with treatment of the gut inflammation. This disease is genetically linked with a histocompatibility antigen found in the blood, called human leukocyte antigen B27 (HLA-B27). Patients with IBD do not have this antigen in excess of that found in the population at large, but it occurs in 80 percent of those with both IBD and ankylosing spondylitis.

Sacroiliitis occurs with ankylosing spondylitis, or by itself. In the latter case, there may be no symptoms, but a pelvic x-ray indicates inflammation of the sacroiliac joints. This form of arthritis progresses independent of the IBD. Symptoms are low back pain, increasing stiffness of the spine, and eventually a stooped posture. The vertebrae become squared, fused, and immobilized as calcified processes fuse along the intervertebral disks. The spine thereby acquires a "bamboo" appearance on x-ray (Figure 16-1). Physiotherapy is essential to minimize crippling pain and deformity.

Unlike colitic arthritis, ankylosing spondylitis is unaffected by colectomy or medical treatment of the IBD. The pain requires analgesia, and narcotic abuse is a worry. Nonsteroidal anti-inflammatory drugs such as aspirin or naproxen (Naprosyn) relieve the pain, but do not alter the course of the disease. Unfortunately, these drugs sometimes seem to exacerbate the accompanying IBD.

Clubbing of the Fingers

Finger clubbing is a curious phenomenon, often associated with a variety of congenital and acquired chronic cardiac and pulmonary diseases. Occasionally it may be found with Crohn's disease, especially when complicated by fistulas or malabsorption.

The fingers and toes are involved, yet there is no pain. The patient may be unaware of the changes. There is softening or sponginess of the base of the nail, loss of the slight angle between

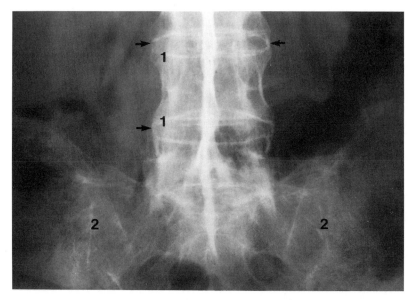

Figure 16-1. Ankylosing spondylitis. Note the rigid, fused vertebra ("bamboo spine") (1), with fusion of the joints around the disks (arrows). The sacroileac joints are obliterated (2). Compare with Figure 27-6.

the nail and long axis of the finger, and sometimes a clawlike curving of the nail.

SKIN MANIFESTATIONS

Erythema Nodosum

Erythema nodosum consists of raised, tender, hot bumps 3 or 4 centimeters in diameter on the shins (Figure 16-2). It is associated with many systemic diseases, including rheumatic fever, tuberculosis, and sarcoidosis, but its justification in this chapter is its occurrence in 3 percent of patients with IBD, especially Crohn's. It is

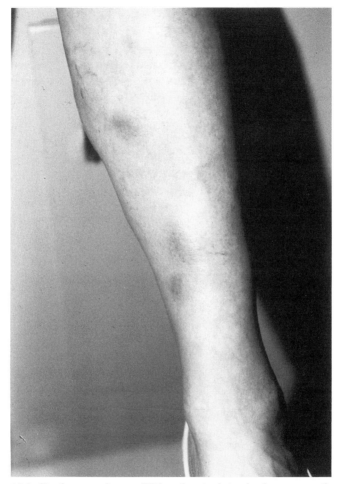

Figure 16-2. Erythema nodosum. With red, raised, tender lumps over the shins, this condition sometimes heralds an attack of IBD.

also frequently accompanied by iritis or colitic arthritis. Like these, it may herald or parallel the attacks of IBD. The nodules subside as the IBD improves, leaving bluish-brown bruises that fade over a few weeks. Treatment of the IBD is effective for erythema nodosum, which itself requires no specific therapy, and leaves no disfigurement or disability. Some patients, warned by erythema nodosum that an attack of IBD is imminent, are able to anticipate therapy.

Pyoderma Gangrenosum

This disfiguring skin disorder is often erroneously thought to be exclusively associated with IBD. In fact, one half of cases are associated with no disease, whereas others are associated with rheumatoid arthritis or chronic malignancies of the blood. The most important connection, however, is with IBD, whose course it may or may not parallel.

The lesion appears to begin as a tiny boil in a hair follicle, but soon develops into a discreet, coinlike lesion, which undermines its purplish rim (Figure 16-3). Usually located on the lower extremity, it may chronically drain pus and be very difficult to treat. The ulcers may be progressive, with the development of sepsis and gangrene (dead tissue) and destruction of the deeper tissues. Disfigurement and rarely fatal septicemia (blood poisoning) may result.

The disease may respond to corticosteroid therapy aimed at the IBD, but other measures are usually necessary. Sterile dressings, dapsone (Avlosulfon), and immunosuppressive drugs such as azathioprine or cyclosporine are often employed. Occasionally a colectomy is performed in an attempt to control the skin disease, but success cannot be guaranteed.

Crohn's Disease of the Skin

Granulomatous lesions may occur around the mouth, anus, or ostomy sites in patients with Crohn's disease. Rarely a Crohn's lesion is seen on the skin, remote from the bowel. Such "metastatic"

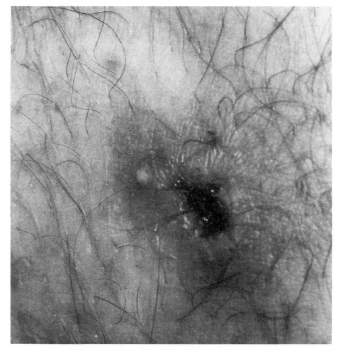

Figure 16-3. Pyoderma gangrenosum.

lesions may occur near the umbilicus. The pathology is similar to that of Crohn's of the bowel, complete with granuloma.

Aphthous Ulcers of the Mouth

Of course, the small, whitish, painful, shallow ulcers commonly known as cankers may occur in the mouth with or without IBD. In IBD, however, they may be plentiful and troublesome. They are similar in appearance to the early lesions of Crohn's disease found in the colon by sigmoidoscopy. One might consider the mouth as part of the gut, but because these lesions are so visible, they are usually considered extraintestinal. The aphthous lesions may appear with the onset of IBD symptoms, and in those receiving large doses of steroids, they may be complicated by a candida infection (thrush). Local treatment with steroid mouth washes (with added nystatin solution if there is candida) is usually helpful. More characteristic Crohn's lesions may also occur in the mouth, such as "cobblestoning," linear ulcers, mucosal tags, and even microscopic granulomas.

LIVER MANIFESTATIONS

Several liver disorders are associated with IBD. Sometimes the liver disturbance is of more consequence than the intestinal disease itself. The prevalence of abnormal liver blood tests among IBD sufferers may be as high as 8 percent. The degree of liver dysfunction and the course of the disease seem to be unrelated to that of the IBD. A simple blood test, the serum alkaline phosphatase, is a sensitive indicator of the presence of the liver disorders that accompany IBD. This enzyme may also be elevated in other diseases, notably of bone, so clinical interpretation is necessary.

SCLEROSING CHOLANGITIS

Recognition of this progressive disease of the bile ducts is important. Although an infrequent complication of IBD, it may prove more difficult to manage than the IBD itself. In this disease there is progressive destruction of the bile ducts both within the liver and between the liver and the duodenum (Figures 16-4 and 1-8). The disease is chronic with a variable course eventually resulting in a biliary cirrhosis. In some cases it may be fatal. It is more common with ulcerative colitis than with Crohn's disease, but its course is independent of either. Sclerosing cholangitis may have no associated disease. It has also been seen to complicate immunodeficiency states such as acquired immunodeficiency syndrome (AIDS).

Most cases are discovered by an elevated alkaline phosphatase, or other liver test abnormality. At this early stage there may be no symptoms. Later, jaundice, itching, weight loss, and the complications of cirrhosis intervene (see the following). The jaundice results from the bile duct obstruction, which prevents the bile pigment bilirubin from escaping to the duodenum, and thence to the feces. Bile salts are produced in the normal liver from cholesterol, and are an important pathway for cholesterol excretion. They also facilitate the absorption of dietary fat from the intestine. With obstruction of these ducts, bile salts, or perhaps some other factor, are increased in the blood and believed to be the cause of the itching.

As the disease progresses, the bile ducts become fibrosed, causing strictures that obstruct, and dilated segments called diverticula occur between the strictures. These abnormalities are seen best by endoscopic retrograde cholangiopancreatography (ERCP) (Figure 16-4), which is the preferred diagnostic procedure (if one can pronounce it!). Liver biopsy may show cirrhosis, or *pericholangitis* (inflammation around the bile ducts), but it does not demonstrate the sclerosing cholangitis.

Itching can be relentless, and the cause of much suffering. Cholestyramine is a resin that, when ingested, binds those bile salts (and perhaps other substances) that do make it to the duodenum, thereby preventing their reabsorption lower in the gut. This reduces the total body stores of these substances, and may relieve the itch. Cholestyramine is of no benefit if bile duct obstruction is complete.

When cirrhosis intervenes, and liver failure threatens, liver transplant is the only treatment. Fortunately, transplantation now affords excellent results.

Chronic Active Hepatitis

This is a chronic disease of liver cells in which are found many autoimmune phenomena. It is occasionally found with IBD. Unlike sclerosing cholangitis, chronic active hepatitis does respond to medical treatment, usually corticosteroids. The result is again cirrhosis, with its many potential complications. Occasionally liver transplant is required. The disease is suspected when liver cell tests, particularly the serum transaminases [aspartate aminotransferase

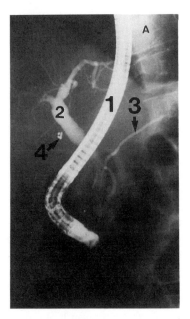

Figure 16-4. (A) This is a normal endoscopic retrograde cholangiopancreatogram (ERCP) in which, through an endoscope (1) placed in the duodenum, radiopaque dye is injected retrograde into the bile duct (2) and pancreatic duct (3). In this case, the gallbladder has been removed, and the clips (4) indicate where the attachment of the gallbladder to the bile ducts was closed.

(AST) or alanine aminotransferase (ALT)] are abnormal. Serum globulins (immune proteins) and tests of disordered immunity, such as the antinuclear factor, are also not normal. The diagnosis is confirmed by liver biopsy.

Cirrhosis

Cirrhosis is the result of many chronic liver diseases, but it may occur apparently without antecedent illness. It may be associated

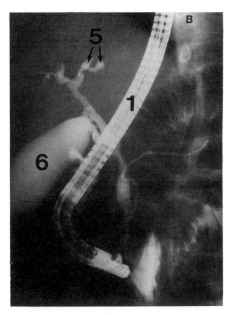

Figure 16-4. (*continued*) (B) This cholangiogram shows destruction of the bile ducts and dilated areas (5) called diverticula, which are characteristic of sclerosing cholangitis. Seen usually with ulcerative colitis, this disease runs an independent course. Sometimes liver transplant is required. In this case, the gallbladder is intact (6).

with IBD through many possible mechanisms. Viral hepatitis (B or C) might be transmitted by a blood transfusion and progress to cirrhosis. Drugs and malnutrition, which damage the liver, may also lead to this common end point, and as we have seen, it may be the last stage of sclerosing cholangitis, or chronic active hepatitis.

Cirrhosis is a scarring of the liver that results in bands of fibrous tissue joining the inflamed areas around the bile ducts, and regeneration of nodules of new but inadequate liver cells. The liver cell destruction is responsible for liver failure, in which the proteins needed for immunity (globulins), maintenance of fluid in the blood vessels (serum albumin), and blood clotting are insufficiently pro-duced. These calamities are compounded when the scarred liver obstructs the portal vein through which blood from the intestines is returned to the heart. This causes fluid to accumulate in the abdomen (ascites), and collateral veins (that bypass the liver) to grow and dilate, especially those around the esophagus. The ascites may be disabling and even become infected. The dilated esophageal veins (varices) may rupture, causing a gastrointestinal hemorrhage.

Gallstones

Gallstones are prone to develop in those with Crohn's disease of the terminal ileum, especially if the ileum is resected. As mentioned previously, the main excretory pathway of cholesterol is via the bile ducts. Cholesterol is insoluble in water and depends on its principal metabolites, the bile salts, to maintain it in solution. These detergent bile salts are excreted with the cholesterol in micel-lar solution into the duodenum. Then, as a conservation measure, they are resorbed sans cholesterol in the terminal ileum, whence they are returned to the liver. If this *enterohepatic* circulation is interrupted by ileal disease or resection, the gallbladder bile becomes deficient in bile salts and supersaturated with choles-terol. Then the cholesterol precipitates, producing cholesterol gall-stones.

Fortunately, most gallstones are asymptomatic and are best left to themselves. If they temporarily or permanently obstruct the bile ducts, however, producing characteristic biliary pain or jaundice, they must be removed. Today there are many choices for their removal: bile salt dissolution, shock wave lithotripsy, and surgical removal of stones or gallbladder. Currently most would choose laparoscopic cholecystectomy for those gallbladder stones that cause severe biliary pain. In this procedure the gallbladder and stones are removed through an endoscope inserted through the abdominal wall. This avoids a major incision and greatly shortens hospitalization. If there are stones in the common bile duct, they are best removed by ERCP, whereby the stone is retrieved via the duodenum using a wire basket. Usually the endoscopist widens the opening (sphincter of Oddi) into the duodenum (see Figure 1-8). This procedure is called a sphincterotomy.

Cholangiocarcinoma

Fortunately rare, cancer of the bile ducts is also associated with IBD, either de novo, or in a case of long-standing sclerosing cholangitis. The symptoms are pain, jaundice, and liver failure. Ultrasound of the liver or ERCP demonstrates the mass around the biliary tree. Sometimes this cancer is difficult to distinguish from sclerosing cholangitis and is found incidentally at the time of liver transplant.

Other Liver Diseases

Many other liver disorders may be associated directly or indirectly with IBD. Fatty infiltration of the liver may occur with protein–calorie malnutrition, and is usually of little consequence, especially if nutrition is restored. Those patients who have required blood transfusions are prone to infection with viral hepatitis, although modern screening of donors should make this a rarity. Abdominal sepsis or obstruction of the common bile ducts with gallstones may cause a liver abscess or bacterial cholangitis. Rarely in ulcerative colitis, the hepatic veins become obstructed, causing blood to congest in the liver (Budd–Chiari syndrome). Drugs such as sulfasalazine may cause a reversible drug hepatitis, and total parenteral nutrition may cause a transient liver dysfunction. Pericholangitis or chronic persistent hepatitis are minor histologic abnormalities that by themselves cause no harm. No list can be complete, for in a common disease such as IBD, coincident liver disease is bound to occur by chance.

OCULAR MANIFESTATIONS

Iritis (uveitis) is the most common eye disease associated with IBD. This is an inflammation in the anterior chamber of the eye characterized by blurred vision, headache, red eye, and pain with light (photophobia). Usually both eyes are affected. Atropine drops are administered to dilate the pupil, and corticosteroid drops reduce the inflammation. Without care, scarring and blindness may result. *Episcleritis* is a lesser eye injury in which inflamed superficial eye tissues cause a burning, red eye. Here again topical steroids are helpful.

RENAL MANIFESTATIONS

Renal Complications of Crohn's Disease

Sometimes the inflammatory mass of ileocecal Crohn's disease extends to the retroperitoneum, where it obstructs the right ureter. This causes the ureter near the kidney to dilate (hydronephrosis) with the risk of renal functional impairment or infection (pyelonephritis). Fistulas from the intestine may burrow their way into the bladder or ureter, producing serious and difficult-to-treat infections in the normally sterile urinary tract. A characteristic symptom of such an enterovesicle fistula is air in the urine (pneumaturia). Urine microscopic examination and culture may detect the infection, but the fistula may be difficult to locate and treat.

Kidney Stones

Kidney stones are common in Crohn's disease. Ileal disease or resection depletes bile salts and permits fat malabsorption. Unabsorbed fatty acids combine with calcium in the gut. This releases oxalate, which is normally bound with the calcium, resulting in increased oxalate absorption from the colon into the blood. In the kidney the oxalate combines with calcium to produce poorly soluble calcium oxalate, which precipitates into a stone in the kidney or ureters.

By another mechanism, individuals with an ileostomy tend to lose fluid and reduce urine volume. The resulting hyperconcentration of urate, a normal urine excretion product, may also produce renal stones.

The consequences of kidney stones may be infection or renal colic. The latter is a severe flank pain radiating to the groin and accompanied by visible or microscopic blood in the urine. Said to be the most severe pain known, it persists for hours, causing its victim to writhe helplessly on the floor. Relief comes when narcotics are given, when the violently contracting ureters give up for a while, or when the stone mercifully passes. Occasionally a urologist must retrieve the stone through a cystoscope (an endoscope passed through the urethra into the bladder).

PANCREATIC MANIFESTATIONS

Pancreatitis seems rare in IBD, and the two may not be significantly related; however, the disease may occur as a complication of investigation or treatment. Pancreatitis may also result from gallstones in the common bile duct. It may complicate in as many as 1 percent of patients undergoing ERCP. Drugs used in the treatment of IBD, such as azathioprine, 6-mercaptopurine (6-MP), and even steroids may rarely cause pancreatitis.

The dominant feature of pancreatitis is severe abdominal pain that pierces through to the back. It may produce serious consequences, such as diabetes, calcium depletion, sepsis, shock, and death. Its rarity in IBD is a blessing.

CARDIOPULMONARY MANIFESTATIONS

A number of rare cardiopulmonary complications of IBD have been reported. These include pericarditis, fibrosing alveolitis, and lung sepsis, but they may only associate by chance, and will not be discussed further here.

HEMATOLOGIC MANIFESTATIONS

The several types of anemia associated with IBD and its treatment have been discussed in Chapters 10 and 14. Blood loss, malabsorption, or dietary lack of nutrients such as iron or folic acid are most important, and of course, there is the anemia of chronic disease. Those anemias due to the 5-aminosalicylic (5-ASA) drugs are discussed in Chapter 20. Loss of protein, malnutrition, or liver damage may result in deficient blood-clotting proteins. Malabsorption of vitamin K in the intestine or failure of its utilization in the liver may cause blood-clotting abnormalities.

THROMBOEMBOLIC MANIFESTATIONS

Pulmonary Embolism

Intravascular blood clotting may have very serious consequences. Clots may develop in the veins of the legs or pelvis of any bedridden patient, especially one with pelvic inflammation such as Crohn's disease. There may, or may not, be swelling of the extremity, but the most serious consequence is dislodgement of the clot from the vein through which it travels via the heart to the lung (pulmonary embolism). The resulting sudden obstruction of a pulmonary artery diverts blood from a segment of the lung and impairs oxygenation. The result may be acute shortness of breath and possible respiratory and cardiac failure and death. The prevention of subsequent events therefore becomes an urgent priority. Anticoagulants are necessary to inhibit clot formation, but are an obvious hazard in a patient with a bleeding gut surface. It is sometimes necessary to install a sieve to catch clots in the main abdominal vein leading to the heart (inferior vena cava).

Pulmonary embolism is best prevented by leg exercises in

bed and early mobilization. Venous thrombosis in the extremity should be suspected when there is calf tenderness or swelling of the limb. An ultrasound device (Doppler) may be used to detect the clot.

Intravascular Clotting and Vasculitis

In active IBD, a hypercoagulable state may exist with a high platelet count and disturbed balance between the clotting and anticlotting proteins in the blood. The situation may be made even more volatile by inflammation in some arteries (vasculitis). In this state, occlusion of the blood supply to vital structures such as the eye or brain may occur. Sometimes the severe inflammation of IBD causes bacteria to travel via the portal vein to the liver. The resulting portal venous infection (portal pyemia) requires urgent application of powerful antibiotics. These terrible consequences are mercifully rare, even in severe IBD.

Amyloidosis

Amyloidosis is a rare disease of arteries occurring in patients with long-standing sepsis and inflammation, and may impair the function of many organs. Affecting predominantly the liver, spleen, and kidneys, it is characterized pathologically by a specific abnormal protein in the tissues. The ultimate result is liver and kidney failure. Opinion is divided over whether excision of the diseased gut alters the course of this unusual complication.

SUMMARY

Inflammatory bowel disease is a disease of the gastrointestinal tract. Nevertheless, there are associated diseases that affect other organs, and that may be of more consequence than the IBD itself. Some, such as colitic arthritis, run a course parallel to that of the underlying intestinal disease and are cured if the IBD is cured, as with colectomy for ulcerative colitis. Others, such as pyoderma gangrenosum or sclerosing cholangitis, acquire a life of their own, uninfluenced by the accompanying IBD. Some, such as kidney stones, gallstones, or hydronephrosis (obstruction of the right ureter), are specific for Crohn's disease, but most occur in both types of IBD. Most IBD sufferers have none of these. Of course, in a disease as common as IBD, other coincident conditions are inevitable, but such coincidence does not prove an association.

CHAPTER SEVENTEEN

IBD and Colon Cancer

Carcinoma of the colon has been recognized as a complication of ulcerative colitis since 1925. Several large centers have reported that after 10 years of disease, 10 percent of their patients developed cancer of the colon. Population studies suggest a lesser risk, but the incidence is such that early recognition and prevention are important issues. The risk of cancer seems to be much less in Crohn's disease, perhaps little greater than that in the general population. The risk in ulcerative colitis increases with the duration and extent of the disease. The recognition of epithelial dysplasia as a harbinger of cancer has led physicians to recommend a surveillance program to ensure its early detection. Such a program involves regular colonoscopies with biopsies, and its costs and benefits incite controversy.

CANCER INCIDENCE IN ULCERATIVE COLITIS

Patients with ulcerative colitis have an increased incidence of colon cancer compared with that of other people. The magnitude of this risk has been the subject of much debate. Reports from large referral centers such as Leeds, London, New York, and the Mayo Clinic indicate that the risk rises sharply after the disease has been present for 10 years. The data are presented in many ways, but these large centers report an incidence of roughly 10 percent after 10 years, 30 to 40 percent after 25 years, and more than 50 percent after 40 years. In contrast, reports from Copenhagen, Czechoslovakia, and a private practice in New York indicate much lower figures. These studies from less selected populations suggest an overall incidence of 0 percent at less than 10 years of disease, about 5 percent at 10 years, and almost 15 percent at 30 years. These differences are more apparent than real, and probably do not represent a geographic variation in risk. Rather, large referral hospitals naturally care for patients with advanced and serious disease, some of whom may already have cancer. Among these selected patients, there is bound to be more cancer. The population and private patient data are likely closer to the true incidence of cancer, because all ulcerative colitis cases are included in the at-risk population, even those with proctitis.

All agree, however, that the risk of cancer is very low when the disease has been present less than 10 years. The risk increases not only with the duration of the disease, but also with the extent of colon involved. Onset of colitis in childhood apparently poses no special risk, but a child has more disease years in which to acquire cancer. Although disease severity or continuous disease are said to be risk factors, it is not unusual for cancer to develop after several years of quiescence. The risk of cancer in ulcerative proctitis seems negligible, but cancer occurs in the rectum of as many as 20 percent of those undergoing ileorectal anastomosis following subtotal colectomy for ulcerative colitis (see Chapter 26). This is one reason that subtotal colectomy with retention of a diseased rectum is seldom performed today.

The long-term ulcerative colitis sufferer is thus haunted by cancer. The risk is too high not to take notice, yet prevention is difficult and controversial. The only sure prevention is timely removal of the colon. There are fewer data available regarding the risk of colon cancer in Crohn's disease, partly because Crohn's colitis was not recognized until 1960. Other cancers, such as lymphoma or carcinoma of the small intestine and anus, may be more common in Crohn's disease. Nevertheless, most experts agree that the risk is much less than that of ulcerative colitis, and prophylaxis is not so big an issue.

CANCER CHARACTERISTICS IN COLITIS

In the general population, colon cancer tends to occur in the 50s or later, whereas that associated with colitis may appear in the 30s. In childhood-acquired ulcerative colitis, it may even strike in the teens. Colon cancers acquired in previously normal colons are readily recognized by barium enema or colonoscopy (Chapter 27). In ulcerative colitis, however, cancer is not so easily seen. The cancer may originate under the epithelial cells and appear as a flat, raised area, or a subtle change in texture of the mucosa. It tends to occur higher in the colon than is the case with spontaneous cancers, and has several sites of origin in about one fourth of cases. This multifocal origin is unusual in ordinary colon cancer. These features make the cancer threat insidious and menacing, and early detection is a challenge; hence, the great interest in dysplasia as a harbinger of cancer, and the notions of cancer surveillance and prophylactic colectomy.

DYSPLASIA

Dysplasia (Figure 17-1) may be best understood as a premalignant change in cells, in this case colon epithelial cells. This histologic phenomenon may also be seen in other cancers, such as those of the lung and cervix. Dysplasia cannot be recognized through endoscopic observation of the colon. Nonetheless, a raised or altered area of mucosa is suspect and should be biopsied. Dysplasia may then be identified by a skilled pathologist.

The histologic features are subtle, and for more information, one should consult a pathology text. Briefly, dysplasia means *unlucky formation* or *abnormal development or growth*. The dysplastic epithelial cells become deeply stained during histologic processing, and the nuclei are disorderly in size, shape, and position within the

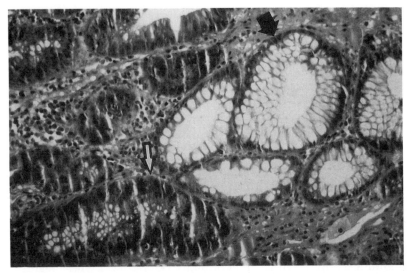

Figure 17-1. Dysplasia. Colon mucosa of a patient with long-standing ulcerative colitis, showing crypts with normal epithelial cells to the right (black arrow), and others demonstrating dysplasia to the left (white arrow). In the latter, the cells have become darkly stained. The dysplastic cell nuclei are large and no longer confined to the base of the cell (compare with Figure 1-2).

cell. Dysplasia is graded as mild, moderate, or severe. Severe dysplasia is sometimes called carcinoma *in situ*. In the presence of acute inflammation, one may see dysplastic lesions, which regress when the colitis is successfully treated. There may be disagreement among pathologists as to the degree, and even the presence of dysplasia; thus, in difficult cases, a second opinion is justified.

About 90 percent of colons removed for colon cancer complicating ulcerative colitis have dysplasia. Most colons in which a biopsy shows dysplasia in the absence of inflammation also contain a cancer; thus, the discovery of colon epithelial dysplasia in a patient with ulcerative colitis is a compelling indication to do a colectomy. There are pitfalls, however. Dysplasia is patchy in distribution, and may be missed by random biopsy. Discovery of dysplasia may occur only after the cancer is well advanced. Occasionally, to everyone's dismay, no cancer may be found at a colectomy prompted by dysplasia.

CANCER SURVEILLANCE IN COLITIS

From the foregoing, the need for an early warning system for cancer becomes obvious. Carcinoembryonic antigen is a tumor antigen associated with colon cancer that can be detected in the blood; however, the test is nonspecific, and we have found increased blood levels of the antigen in nearly 20 percent of patients with inflammatory bowel disease (IBD). One of the features of ulcerative colitis is bleeding, so testing the stool for occult traces of blood is equally useless. Because the lesions are flat and submucosal, and because the colon is already distorted by the colitis, a barium enema is of little value in early cancer detection. Thus colonoscopy with multiple biopsies in search of dysplasia is the only practical detection method available. Even here there are difficulties. Colonoscopy is a costly and uncomfortable test. Who should have it and how often? Further, even the most thorough colonoscopic surveillance will fail to discover some cancers before they are too advanced to cure.

Most agree that the cancer risk is negligible in ulcerative proctitis or disease of less than 10 years' duration. It is greatest in long-standing pancolitis. It is commonly recommended to commence annual colonoscopies in such patients after 10 years of disease. Biopsies are taken every 10 centimeters throughout the colon. If dysplasia is found in the absence of inflammation, and confirmed by a repeat test 6 to 12 weeks later, a colectomy is recommended. Dysplasia in an endoscopically observed lesion is particularly worrisome [dysplasia-associated lesion or mass (DALM)]. Such a regimen should lead to the early detection and cure of the cancer, yet sadly the results of surgery in such cases are little different from those in ordinary colon cancer in which, depending on the stage of the tumor, the 5-year survival rate is about 50 percent. This leads to much debate regarding the surveillance policy. Some believe that the cost is too great, and the benefits, too low. Perhaps one colonoscopy at 10 years is enough? If dysplasia is not found, exponents of this policy say no more testing is required. Most would be unhappy with this, but the tests may not need to be repeated every year. Others favor a prophylactic colectomy after 10 years or so depending on the severity of the colitis, the risk factors, and individual preference. It is important that a patient understand these dilemmas, for he or she ultimately must decide.

PROPHYLACTIC COLECTOMY

Some Europeans recommend removal of the colon when the perceived cancer risk is high; thus, patients with pancolitis are offered colectomy by 20 years. In Copenhagen, about one third of those with ulcerative colitis had a colectomy by 18 years. The decision becomes easier if the colitis itself is troublesome, or other complications threaten. Even in remission, the colon may be so rigid and narrowed that normal function can no longer be anticipated. Some argue that modern surgical techniques provide for a virtually risk-free colectomy. New techniques also permit the fashioning of an ileal pouch as a new rectum, so that the need of an ileostomy is obviated (see Chapter 26). One thing is certain: without a colon, one can no longer have ulcerative colitis or colon cancer.

SUMMARY

Patients with ulcerative colitis are at risk for developing cancer of the colon. This risk becomes apparent after 10 years of colitis and increases with the duration and extent of the disease. The risk seems much less in Crohn's disease. Early detection of cancer in ulcerative colitis should lead to curative resection, but there are many difficulties. Colonoscopy and biopsy in search of the premalignant lesion (dysplasia) is the only available surveillance method; however, colonoscopy is expensive and uncomfortable, biopsies may miss the lesion, and dysplasia may be found too late to ensure a cure.

Nevertheless, annual colonoscopies are commonly recommended after 10 years, and the discovery of persistent dysplasia in the absence of acute inflammation should prompt early colectomy. Because this policy is not foolproof, many physicians tend to recommend early colectomy to obviate the risk. Such a decision is easier when the colitis itself is troublesome, but cancer, it should be remembered, may occur after years of quiescent disease.

CHAPTER EIGHTEEN

Psychological Factors and Quality of Life

Like many of you, I thought my life was over. But I learned that you can come back. Maybe at first you don't think you will, but believe me you're wrong. You can!

Rolf Benirschke, 1986

Ulcerative colitis and Crohn's disease, first recognized early in this century, are of unknown cause. This etiologic void has led to many theories. An early concept was that these diseases, especially colitis, were psychogenic; that is, they resulted from repressed psychological conflict or maladaption to stress. The theory held that a predisposing personality associated with a biologic cause led to clinical expression of the disease. For many years prior to the development of effective therapy, there was a strongly held notion that one could identify a colitis personality, which was somehow responsible for the disease. This concept seems simplistic today, but it is still possible that stress influences timing of the illness in a biologically susceptible person. Only recently have we come to see psychological problems more as a result of or coincident to the disease than as its cause. Nevertheless, the earlier concept of a colitis personality has had some damaging effect. It has stigmatized some patients with inflammatory bowel disease (IBD) and could cause discrimination and even some reluctance to care for them among health care workers.

To deal with these issues, it is first necessary to consider the effects of psychosocial problems on the disease. More important, it becomes obvious that we must consider the effects of the disease on the person physically *and* psychologically. The quality of life (QOL) is an important consideration if we are to assess the impact of the disease on someone. Whether or not a person is disabled over the long term depends as much on his or her psychosocial status as on the disease itself. Once these relationships are understood, we can better comprehend the issues of disability and insurability.

EFFECT OF PSYCHOSOCIAL FACTORS ON IBD

Many IBD patients and their physicians believe that stress is important in the generation of disease activity. This may be true, but it is difficult to prove. One prospective, 2-year trial failed to show that increased stress or depressed mood preceded the exacerbations of the disease. Psychological factors appear to loom large in some other diseases, such as peptic ulcer or neurogenic dermatitis, but in IBD it has proven difficult to distinguish between stress as a medium for increased gut inflammation and stress that impairs one's ability to cope with or tolerate the symptoms.

Psychosomatic medicine was a popular theory with a previous generation of physicians, led by Engel. This concept held that disruption of the person's psychosocial environment impairs his or her ability to cope. Thus psychosocial factors do not in themselves cause IBD, but rather contribute to its onset in genetically susceptible individuals. This idea was largely misunderstood, because some insisted that IBD, particularly ulcerative colitis, is actually caused by psychological factors. Placed in proper context, psychosocial factors deserve consideration in the interaction of a patient with his physical illness. Moreover, perhaps through psychological effects on the immune system, the actual pathologic process may be altered. Those who doubt this should be aware that IBD patients not responding to maximal medical therapy frequently improve with little change in medication when admitted to the hospital. Such temporary removal from day-to-day concerns seems therapeutic.

Earlier data suggesting that colitis victims suffer a dependent relationship with a domineering parent resulted from psychiatric assessments of a group of subjects selectively referred because of their apparent psychologic maladjustment. Most IBD patients do not see a psychiatrist. These data are retrospective and are uncontrolled by comparisons to normals, other IBD sufferers, or psychiatric patients. Similar criticisms apply to data suggesting that IBD patients have dependent, immature personalities and are overly sensitive to interpersonal rejection. Most physicians would reject this on the basis of observations of their own patients. Furthermore, there is no evidence that people with psychiatric illness are prone to develop IBD.

There is some experimental evidence that stress may alter the immune system and thereby impair resistance to infection or exacerbate local inflammation. One study indicates that stressful life events are associated with symptoms, but not rectal inflammation in ulcerative colitis; however, high levels of perceived stress predict rectal inflammation but not symptoms. Hence, it remains possible that stress might trigger the onset or an exacerbation of the disease. Clinically, such a phenomenon has been observed in patients with the irritable bowel syndrome, but as mentioned previously, not in IBD. It seems likely to be more important that, in IBD, psychosocial factors, stress, and psychiatric illness result from the disease, or impair one's ability to adapt to illness.

EFFECT OF IBD ON THE PERSON

The separation of psychology from the premises of biology is purely artificial, because the human psyche lives in indissoluble union with the body.

Carl Jung (1875–1961)

There can be no doubt that IBD may cause significant disturbance of a person's psychological and social well-being. Particularly in Crohn's disease, there is a high incidence of major depression. All sufferers inevitably have some psychological fallout. Lengthy presence of abdominal pain, the need to catalogue all public toilets in range of one's travels, or to confine oneself to the convenience of his or her own bathroom can profoundly affect one's social life. Remember, IBD usually begins in youth when personality and social skills are still developing. The malaise of the illness and the need for surgery may cause profound social disruption.

Special problems may damage the IBD patient's body image. Fear of an ostomy is very prevalent, yet often unjustified. In adolescents, delayed puberty, growth retardation, and inability to be as active in sports may spawn lifelong effects. Here aggressive therapy, even surgery is indicated (Chapter 26). Severe perianal disease, especially a rectovaginal fistula, can have devastating psychosexual implications.

Many young people fear for the future. "Will I get married?" "Can I have children?" "Is a steady job possible?" "Does my disease, my ileostomy, my fistula, my perianal abscess make me socially and sexually unacceptable?" These are almost universal, but not often stated questions that haunt the young person with IBD. Individual reactions to these dilemmas are as varied as the human mind permits. Some deny their disease and rebelliously miss appointments, or disregard medical instructions. Others may become depressed or withdrawn. In one study, 30 percent of those with Crohn's disease concealed their disease from their employers. Even contemplation of suicide is not uncommon.

For most IBD patients, a far more optimistic outlook is justified. Timely counsel is therefore very important. Those concerns related to sex and reproduction are further discussed in the next chapter. Inflammatory bowel disease, indeed any illness, has an important impact on psychosocial well-being. Before we explore how this interacts with the physical manifestations of disease to affect QOL, we must consider one other component of the psychosocial–sexual– physical stew, illness behavior.

ILLNESS BEHAVIOR

Illness behavior refers to the manner in which an individual perceives, evaluates, and reacts to symptoms. People respond to any illness in a variety of ways depending on their attitudes and their psychosocial situation. An IBD patient may delay medical attention if he or she feels that the symptoms are of no consequence, is concerned about cost, believes complaining is a weakness, is reluctant to take time off work, or fears the consequences of the consultation, such as drugs and x-rays. Conversely, a similar patient may seek attention if a symptom is new, or if he or she thinks it might do harm, has a dependent relationship with the doctor, or comes from a family where great attention is paid to illness. Extreme examples of the latter might become labeled hypochondriacs.

The seeking of medical attention and intervention may be influenced by all sorts of seemingly extraneous factors. In western cultures, women are more likely than men to consult, whereas in India, the opposite is true. Some racial groups tend to respond dramatically to pain, but Anglo-Saxons are culturally conditioned to deny it or "bear it." In the Third World, diarrhea may be so common that it is not considered an illness. These differences are important but manageable if the physician–patient relationship is functioning properly.

The consequences are much more damaging if a person perceives any benefit from being sick. Some may assume a sick role with minor provocation because they learned such behavior early in life; that is, minor illnesses permitted them to stay home from school or receive special favors or gifts. Even minor pains or bowel disruption may be used, perhaps subconsciously, to avoid work, family obligations, or stressful situations, or to gratify a dependent relationship with a relative or health care worker. Depressed persons also express exaggerated physical complaints. Hypochondriacs amplify apparently mild dysfunction into worries about serious illness.

One of the most destructive determinants of inappropriate illness behavior is the existence of secondary-gain possibilities, such as disability benefits. Most IBD patients want and are able to work most of the time; therefore, pre-existing disability insurance is an important component of their well-being. Such insurance is difficult to obtain once IBD is established (see the following). Once a person perceives his happiness to be greater on long-term disability than on the work force, however, his or her perception of illness may be altered. Very often the interpretation of illness and disability in this very small group of patients is at variance with that of others, particularly insurance companies, and can negatively affect medical care and rehabilitation. No one, of course, can measure pain, and even the quality of bowel habit is usually in the eye of the beholder. Exaggerated complaints can generate unnecessary tests and treatments that may do psychological or physical harm. Those caring for the patient may find themselves in an awkward position as arbiters of disability. The care-giver may feel that long-term disability benefits are unnecessary, even harmful, but it is difficult to deny a patient's complaints. Thus, continuing uncertainty conflicts with good, objective medical care. Resolution of this conflict of interest requires patience, compassion, and wisdom by all concerned.

QUALITY OF LIFE

Because of the protean manifestations of IBD and its unpredictable course, it is difficult to measure the degree of disease. Yet such measurement is essential to the assessment of the efficacy of therapy, both in clinical trials and in practice. In order to provide a yardstick of disease activity, several scales employing objective measures have been developed. The most famous of these is the Crohn's Disease Activity Index (CDAI), developed for the National Cooperative Crohn's Disease Study and described in Chapter 24 (Table 24-1). This index and others like it evaluate several physical parameters to arrive at a score that reflects disease activity. When recorded by an independent observer, the index is a comparatively objective measure of disease before and after treatment, or between patients. Because ongoing direct observation of the diseased gut is impractical, an activity index is indispensable in the testing of drug therapy.

The CDAI, however, does not measure how a patient functions with the disease, or how he feels about it. In this context, it should be remembered that treatments themselves may adversely affect function and feelings. Drugs such as steroids or an ileostomy may be fair trade-offs for the physical disease, but their negative effects on QOL may be self-defeating. Therefore, many physicians have come to believe that health-related QOL measures (HRQOL) are as

TABLE 18-1
Disease-related Concerns in IBD

Uncertain nature of my disease	Attractiveness
Effects of medication	Having access to quality medical care
Energy level	Dying early
Having surgery	Intimacy
Having an ostomy bag	Loss of sexual drive
Being a burden on others	Feeling alone
Loss of bowel control	Financial difficulties
Developing cancer	Ability to perform sexually
Ability to achieve full potential	Passing the disease to others
Producing unpleasant odors	Feeling "dirty" or "smelly"
Feelings about my body	Being treated as different
Pain or suffering	Ability to have children
Feeling out of control	

important as physical measures in the assessment of disease or treatment impact. To be sure, how we function is greatly influenced by the psychosocial factors discussed earlier in this chapter, but because a happy, functioning person should be the primary objective of care, anything that affects function or attitude is relevant.

Using questionnaires such as the Sickness Impact Scale and a Rating Form of IBD concerns (Table 18-1), Drossman and his associates examined a group of patients, mainly from North Carolina (63 ulcerative colitis, 87 Crohn's) who represent a clinical population. Data from these patients suggested that:

1. Patients with IBD experience moderate functional impairment, more in the social and psychological than in the physical dimension.
2. Patients with Crohn's disease report more psychosocial dysfunction than do patients with colitis.
3. Patients with IBD express greatest concerns about having surgery, decrease in energy, and body image issues, such as having an ostomy bag.
4. Functional status and patients' concerns correlate better with

other measures of health status and health care utilization than with the physician's rating of disease activity.

Drossman also studied a group comprising 997 members of the Crohn's and Colitis Foundation of America (CCFA). Of these 320 had ulcerative colitis and 671 had Crohn's disease. Unlike the first group, these subjects were volunteers and were perhaps not exactly representative of all IBD patients. In any case, their responses raise several additional issues. First, despite the symptoms and complications attributed to IBD, the health status of this population was generally good. This may be due to a better coping style among these volunteers. Supporting this, Binder reports that among all the IBD patients of Copenhagen, about one half were symptom free in any one year, and another one fourth were not severely affected. Second, those Crohn's disease patients with greater disability appear to have greater symptom severity. Both psychosocial and physical health variables are related to the number of physician visits, whereas physical health variables accounted for hospitalization and surgery.

Greater IBD concerns appear to be related to disease severity, female gender, and lower educational status. Therefore, education directed at women and the poor with the disease may pay the greatest dividend in lessening concern and improving QOL. Not surprisingly, fear of cancer was prevalent in ulcerative colitis, whereas pain and suffering, concern about being a burden to others, financial difficulties, and energy loss seemed more characteristic concerns in Crohn's disease.

Using direct interview rather than a questionnaire, Farmer and associates studied QOL in 164 outpatients, 94 with ulcerative colitis, and 70 with Crohn's disease. They too observed that the QOL was better in ulcerative colitis than in Crohn's, but further noted that in both, it was better than that found in two other chronic, low-mortality diseases, multiple sclerosis and rheumatoid arthritis. Those who had surgery indicated a lower QOL, but that may be a reflection of disease severity (see Chapter 26).

Binder found that 122 patients with ulcerative colitis were similar to age-matched controls in regard to marriage, financial status, and incidence of severe family, sexual, or drug problems. A companion study of 108 Crohn's patients also revealed a very good QOL. The unemployment rate was the same as that of controls. The IBD patients tended to have better education and socioeconomic status, which may have helped them cope. Despite these findings, both groups of IBD patients felt their disease strained their personal and professional lives. Among the Crohn's disease patients, 3 percent were on a disability pension.

The foregoing data confirm that, all things considered, for most IBD patients the disease-related QOL is good. Nonetheless, a patient's psychosocial concerns are as important as physical symptoms in measuring the impact of the disease and should be part of any assessment or management strategy, either in clinical trials or in real life. Questions such as those implied in Table 18-1 may expose inappropriate concerns. Education and explanation may dissipate those concerns and have a salutary effect on a patient's QOL.

INSURANCE

Many IBD patients report difficulty in obtaining insurance. Nonetheless an informal survey of members of the Canadian Association of Ileitis and Colitis (CFIC) indicates that of those who applied for life insurance, two thirds were successful. Those with Crohn's disease tended to be charged a higher premium, however. Smokers were more likely to be rejected. It is possible that many who should apply, don't, and others, once rejected, never try again. Modern IBD death rates differ little, if any, from those of the rest of the population; thus, it should be possible for most patients to eventually be insured, provided there is no other risk factor, such as hypertension or illicit drug use.

Life insurance is a very competitive business, which is subject to international trade pressures. Insurance companies want our business, but of course also wish to minimize risk. A recent discussion group of physicians and insurance industry representatives sponsored by the CFIC produced the following advice for IBD patients wishing life insurance. First, be persistent. If rejected by one company, try another. If rejected when ill, try again after a period of remission, say 2 to 4 years. Mortality is thought to be higher early in the disease, so early rejection may convert to later acceptance. If initially charged an extra premium, ask to have this reviewed once in remission a few years. An insurance company cannot increase your rates, but might lower them to keep your business. Eliminate other risk factors, especially smoking. Insurance companies are reassured by regular physician check-ups, especially if the clinical report is good. For obvious reasons, applications for either trifling or very large amounts of money invite rejection. Despite the foregoing, those with both small- and large-bowel disease, those with extensive jejunal disease that threatens nutrition, or those within a year or two of surgery are considered high risk. Even here, risk appears to be decreasing, and persistence may pay off over time. Obviously, those eligible for group life insurance are at an advantage.

Insurance against disability or drug costs is another matter. In IBD, the likelihood of payouts is high, and few companies will entertain the risk, especially outside of groups. Here again, it pays to shop around. Chances improve if the patient is in a group, in remission, or has had a colectomy for ulcerative colitis. When changing jobs, an IBD patient should take care that any insurance benefits are portable, or at least available to him or her in the new employer's group plan. If not, lack of coverage should be weighed against the benefits of the new job.

SUMMARY AND CONCLUSIONS

There is little evidence that psychological factors are the cause of IBD, although they could alter the disease in biologically susceptible people. They may, however, greatly affect one's ability to cope with the manifestations of the disease and hence bear greatly on employment and the QOL. The dignity and fortitude with which most IBD patients endure their illness is impressive to the medical observer. As a result, the QOL in IBD, especially ulcerative colitis, is good relative to that of other chronic diseases. Yet for some, psychosocial factors are very troubling, and may generate illness behavior, disability, and a deteriorating QOL. In some of these patients, a QOL assessment might expose misapprehensions and concerns about the disease that, when properly dealt with, might improve functioning. The prospects for marriage, children, employment, and even life insurance are relatively good. Despite periods of severe disease activity, patients should be reassured by these facts.

The last word here belongs to Rolf Benirschke, star place-kicker for the San Diego Chargers. At the peak of his football career, Rolf acquired colitis. He lost 50 pounds and was near death before undergoing emergency surgery. Two years later, equipped with an ileostomy, he kicked a playoff game-winning overtime field goal against the Miami Dolphins. Another attack sidelined him again, but again his skill, courage, and the support of family and friends permitted him to fashion another "great comeback." Since then, in cooperation with the Crohn's and Colitis Foundation of America (CCFA), Rolf has promoted the Great Comebacks program with annual awards for equally determined people with IBD. No IBD sufferer should feel that a great comeback is beyond his or her reach.

> Maybe at first you think you never will [come back], but believe me, you're wrong. You can!

CHAPTER NINETEEN

Sex and Reproduction with IBD

Inflammatory bowel disease (IBD) strikes its victims during their adolescence or reproductive years. Quite apart from the pain and malaise of the disease itself, for the patient there is an often unstated worry about his or her marital and reproductive future. There is no doubt that severe symptoms of IBD may physically deter one from engaging in sex, or bearing children in the short term. Remissions are usual, however, and in ulcerative colitis, at least, a curative colectomy is always at hand. The physical impediments are seldom permanent, but psychological and social difficulties, fed by ignorance and needless worry, may trouble young people with this disease. Adolescents face enough problems maturing in today's atmosphere of easy divorce and sexually transmitted diseases, without carrying the added baggage of IBD. Frank discussion of sexual issues with a physician or nurse, strong family support, and an informed and caring partner or spouse are special requirements of the young IBD sufferer. The bottom line is that there can be sex and reproduction in almost every IBD patient's future.

BODY IMAGE

Chronic illness delays maturation and causes weight loss and a pallid, sickly complexion. During exacerbations of IBD, such appearances, compounded by the effects of steroids, cause patients to feel unattractive to the opposite sex. A young person with IBD should be reassured that he or she will not always appear ill. Remissions are possible with drugs, although sometimes slow to achieve. Occasionally surgery is required. When the disease is eventually controlled, the patient feels better, and the desire for sex returns, along with weight and a healthy complexion. Delayed maturation in an adolescent is an indication for early surgery. The young, however, are "now" people, and patience while one awaits a remission is almost too much to ask. This is why counseling, emotional support, and understanding are so important. In ulcerative proctitis, or mild cases of IBD, there are few external manifestations of the disease, and these difficulties must not be considered inevitable.

Disfigurement from the disease is especially troublesome. Some of the extraintestinal complications of IBD, such as pyoderma gangrenosum or arthritis, impair one's body image, but these may be minimized with specialist care. Colitis patients considering colectomy worry about the unnatural appearance of an ileostomy and how it may affect a sexual partner. Such a patient should be reassured that he or she will feel so much better with their colon removed, that an ileostomy will not deter him or her, or an understanding partner. The usual outcome is marriage, sex, and children (although not necessarily in that order). Added comfort has accompanied the development of new ileal anal pouches that obviate the need for an ileostomy (Chapter 26).

Such comfort may be less convincing to a patient with Crohn's disease, for which no such surgical cure is at hand. Dependence on drugs or recurrences after surgery are therefore common dilemmas. Nonetheless, skillful medical and surgical management should ensure frequent remissions during which sex and reproduction can be normal. Most troublesome is severe perianal disease. This can seem to be an insurmountable impediment to sexual relations. Fistula from gut to vagina or bladder may for a time make intercourse at once physically and psychologically impossible.

Even when in remission, a patient may feel too deformed to even try. Counseling by nurse or doctor of both patient and partner may help, and discussion with other similarly afflicted patients may be constructive.

It is important to keep sight of the bottom line. Although temporarily out of action, the IBD patient can look forward to a future of sex and children. Good medical care, education, understanding, and patience all contribute to this future.

FERTILITY

Effect of the Disease

When the patient is ill, conception is unlikely. A woman's menstruation is often suppressed for the duration; however, the normal cycle returns with disease remission, and conception is again possible. Studies in the United States and Britain have found that fertility, that is, the ability to conceive, is similar in women with ulcerative colitis and the normal population. About 10 percent of both groups are infertile, and in 40 percent of these it is the male who is at fault. There does appear to be some reduction in fertility among women with Crohn's disease, but the magnitude is uncertain. Failure to conceive may be due to several factors beyond the disease itself. Libido may be suppressed. Nutrition may be undercorrected. Pelvic IBD may damage the reproductive apparatus, or create a psychological as well as physical barrier to sexual relations. Some patients may decide they do not wish a family, or may be advised (I think unwisely) not to conceive. Of course, women with IBD may be infertile from other causes, and deserve the same workup in a fertility clinic as those without IBD. The disease should not, in itself, be an indication for a therapeutic abortion.

Effect of Medication

Sulfasalazine depresses the production of sperm in males, and alters the appearance of those that are produced. Fortunately, these return to normal when the drug is withdrawn. The newer 5-amino-salicylic acid (5-ASA) compounds, which contain no sulfonamide, do not seem to have this effect (see Chapter 20).

The impact of prednisone and the immunosuppressive drugs on conception has been insufficiently studied. When these drugs are employed, the activity of the disease itself may depress fertility, making it difficult to identify a drug effect. As discussed later, on principle it is best when conception occurs in the absence of medication.

Effect of Surgery

A total colectomy with resection of the rectum puts men at risk for impotence or other sexual dysfunction. With expert technique, such a risk should be much less than 10 percent. With the new anal pouch–ileal anastomosis, there is even less chance of damage to the sacral nerves, and hence, less risk of infertility. Some women experience painful intercourse after pelvic surgery, especially with the pouch procedure. There is no evidence that the surgery impairs fertility in women (see Chapter 26).

PREGNANCY

Effect of IBD on Pregnancy

As a general rule, it is best to become pregnant when the IBD is quiescent and the drugs are safely withdrawn. Nevertheless, the effect of IBD on pregnancy is less than one might expect. In particular, ulcerative colitis seldom interferes with fetal survival. Spontaneous abortions, prematurity, deformities, and stillbirths are no more common than in the normal population. The presence of active disease during conception might increase the risk of a preterm delivery, and maybe low birth weight. Of course complications of colitis, such as toxic magacolon, or other need for urgent surgery, are bound to be a threat to the lives of both mother and child.

Fortunately, these are very rare. Clearly careful follow-up and care of the IBD during pregnancy is important.

The presence of Crohn's disease also seems to have little effect on the outcome of pregnancy. Indeed one American study even suggests that the increased attention afforded such pregnancies improves the outlook. Nevertheless, such optimism must be tempered in cases in which the Crohn's was active at conception or when it manifests for the first time during pregnancy. Severe exacerbations of the disease, or the need to operate on a pelvic complication, can only increase fetal risk.

In most cases of pregnancy in IBD, vaginal delivery is feasible. This is true even after total colectomy or other abdominal surgery. The principal exception is pelvic Crohn's disease. There are cases of rectovaginal fistula occurring postdelivery, so severe pelvic inflammation may provoke a caesarian section. Another exception may be the fashioning of an ileal pouch with anal anastomosis following total colectomy for ulcerative colitis. In one series of 20 healthy deliveries after such surgery, 9 were by caesarian section (Chapter 26).

The severely ill patient with suppressed menstruation is naturally protected from conception. In others with active IBD, it is simply good sense to await a quiescent period, preferably without drug requirement, and to ensure that nutrition is optimal. It is also wise to ensure a dialogue between the physician caring for the patient with IBD, and an obstetrician skilled in increased-risk pregnancies. With these precautions, the overall outlook for a pregnancy in a woman with IBD seems little different from normal.

Effect of Pregnancy on IBD

Inflammatory bowel disease behaves similarly in the pregnant and nonpregnant state. When inactive at conception, the disease has a 75 percent chance of remaining so throughout pregnancy. When disease does manifest, it is generally within the first 3 to 6 months. If active at the beginning, the disease tends to worsen throughout gestation. Older reports suggest that first attacks or relapses were more severe during pregnancy or the postpartum period. Modern studies indicate that this is not now the case. No doubt the realization that the 5-ASA compounds and prednisone could be safely administered during pregnancy has led to better disease control. In difficult Crohn's disease, timely surgery prior to conception may achieve a remission and permit a safe pregnancy. Of course, total colectomy for ulcerative colitis virtually removes the risk.

In the individual case it is impossible to predict the effect of a pregnancy on the disease; neither is the outcome of a previous pregnancy a safe predictor of the next. In general, however, it seems that the chance of an IBD relapse during pregnancy is the same as if pregnancy had not occurred.

Investigations during Pregnancy

When the disease worsens or begins during pregnancy, some investigation may be required. In ulcerative colitis, stool cultures, blood tests, and sigmoidoscopy usually suffice. Colonoscopy may be performed in early pregnancy if deemed necessary to determine the extent of disease, or detect proximal Crohn's colitis. Usually it may be deferred. Ultrasound is safe and may help assess both disease and fetus, but x-rays should be avoided, especially in the first 3 months. Of course, caution must be suspended in an emergency such as a suspected perforation or obstruction.

Treatment during Pregnancy

The principles of treatment of BID during pregnancy are similar to those in the nonpregnant state. Hydration, nutrition, correction of anemia, and psychological and physical rest are primary objectives. In some cases, intravenous infusion of fluid, and enteral or parenteral (intravenous) nutrition may be necessary. Severe complications may even require surgery.

Because sulfasalazine crosses the placenta and appears in

minute quantities in the breast milk, there was concern that the drug might harm the fetus. This worry has been dispelled by several studies. The use of the newer 5-ASA products in pregnancy has been studied less, but they should be at least as safe, since they do not include a sulfonamide. Most experts recommend their use when required during pregnancy. In ulcerative colitis, maintenance of a prophylactic 5-ASA drug through pregnancy is a matter of personal choice. Despite indications that the drug is very safe, on principle, some will withdraw the drug prior to conception. If sulfasalazine is used, ample folic acid should be given to overcome the drug's folate antagonism.

Although it is difficult to separate the effects of drugs from those of the disease they are designed to treat, studies indicate that prednisone does not harm the fetus. This may in part be due to the fact that prednisone does not cross the placental barrier. As in the case of any acute stress, those on chronic steroid treatment must have the dose increased during labor and delivery.

Most would agree that immunosuppressive drugs are contraindicated in pregnancy. Despite a small study showing safety of azathioprine and the low incidence of fetal harm in renal transplant patients, I would not recommend this or any other immunosuppressive during or after conception. Some would even consider accidental conception while on such a drug to be an indication for a therapeutic abortion. Metronidazole has the potential for fetal harm and should also be avoided in pregnancy.

SUMMARY

The IBD sufferer's reproductive life may be threatened by the disfiguring nature of the disease, infertility, or inability on the part of a woman to sustain a pregnancy. In most cases the body-image impairment due to active disease or its treatment are not permanent. Remissions permit normal maturation and sexual activity. Even perianal disease or an ileostomy need not prevent sex and marriage. When a woman is severely ill, menstruation is suppressed, and conception is impossible. Fertility returns with remission. If quiescent at conception, IBD should not adversely affect the pregnancy, and remission continues throughout in most cases. Attacks, usually occur within the first few months. They likely occur with the same frequency whether the person is pregnant or not. Prednisone and the 5-ASA compounds, however, appear to be safe in pregnancy. Nevertheless, it seems prudent to discontinue all drugs before conception and during pregnancy. Spontaneous abortion, prematurity, deformities, and stillbirths seem no different from those expected in the normal population, although the outlook might be better in ulcerative colitis than in Crohn's disease. For most IBD patients, the future usually includes sex, marriage, and children.

PART FIVE

Treatments and Investigations

CHAPTER TWENTY

5-ASA

5-Aminosalicylic acid (5-ASA) is a salicylate related to aspirin. It is topically (locally) effective in the management of ulcerative colitis and Crohn's disease. Salicylazosulfapyridine (sulfasalazine) is a drug that consists of a 5-ASA molecule joined to a sulfapyridine molecule by an azo bond (Figure 20-1). The drug was developed 50 years ago in Sweden as a treatment for rheumatoid arthritis, but, in the course of clinical trials, it was noticed that bowel symptoms improved in those patients who also had ulcerative colitis (see Chapter 4). It has since found steady employment for the treatment of that disease. As we shall see, 5-ASA is the active principle. The newer oral and rectal preparations represent attempts by the pharmaceutical industry to find alternatives to sulfapyridine as a vehicle to deliver 5-ASA to the inflamed bowel.

The following is a discussion of sulfasalazine and its newer 5-ASA alternatives, with attention to the nature of the drugs, their action in inflammatory bowel disease (IBD), and their unwanted effects. The 5-ASA preparations available in Canada are summarized in Table 20-1. Most are, or soon will be, obtainable in the United States. The choice of drug is made on the basis of site of release of 5-ASA, side-effects, and cost (Table 20-2). The efficacy of sulfasalazine in IBD is scientifically established; however, our knowl-

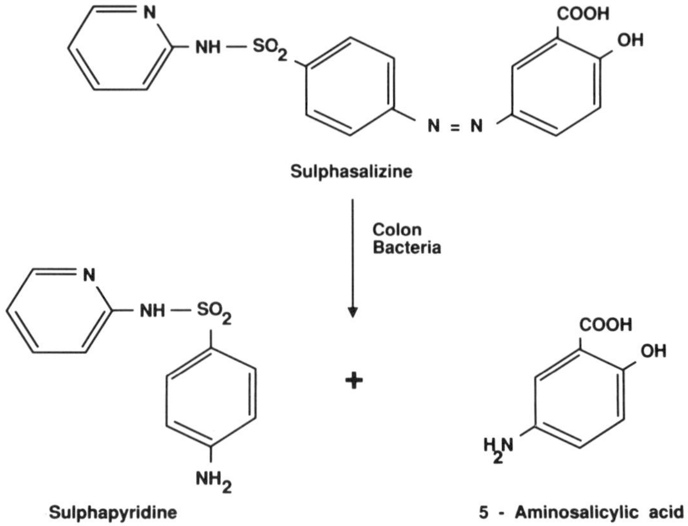

Figure 20-1. The azo bond of sulfasalazine is cleaved by colon bacteria, releasing sulfapyridine and 5-aminosalicylic acid (5-ASA).

TABLE 20-1
5-ASA Preparations

Drug	Brand name	Means of delivery	Activity
Sulfasalazine	Salazopyrin Azulfidine	Bacterial degradation	Colon
Olsalazine	Dipentum	Bacterial degradation	Colon
Mesalamine 5-ASA	Asacol	Embedded in eudragit S, dispersed at pH 7	Colon
Mesalamine 5-ASA	Salofalk Mesasal Claversal	Embedded in eudragit L, dispersed at pH 6	Colon and ileum
	Salofalk enema	Topical	Left colon
	Salofalk suppository	Topical	Anorectum
Mesalamine 5-ASA	Pentasa	Ethylcellulose coated, slow release	Small bowel and colon

TABLE 20-2
Cost of 5-ASA Preparations[a]

Drug	Brand name	Unit strength	Cost/ unit	Dose/ day	Cost/ month[b]
Sulfasalazine	Salazopyrin	500 mg	$0.18	4 g	$53.15
		500 mg[c]	$0.27	4 g	$74.75
	Generic	500 mg	$0.11	4 g	$33.35
Olsalazine	Dipentum	250 mg	$0.51	2 g	$132.35
Mesalamine	Asacol	400 mg	$0.53	2 g	$89.45
	Mesasal	500 mg	$0.58	2 g	$79.55
	Salofalk	250 mg	$0.38	2 g	$101.15
		500 mg	$0.53	2 g	$73.55
	Pentasa	250 mg	$0.35	2 g	$93.95
		500 mg	$0.62	2 g	$84.35
5-ASA suppositories	Salofalk	250 mg	$0.69	1 g	$92.75
		500 mg	$1.14	1 g	$78.35
5-ASA enemas	Salofalk	4 gram/60 ml	$6.25	4 g	$197.45

[a]1993 cost in $Canadian. $US rate approximately × .80.
[b]Pharmacy fee included.
[c]Enteric coated.

edge of the therapeutic value of the newer drugs is largely extrapolated from the sulfasalazine experience.

SULFASALAZINE
(SALICYLAZOSULFAPYRIDINE)

With the introduction of less toxic 5-ASA pharmaceutical preparations, the use of sulfasalazine is declining. Nevertheless, there are still situations in which it is the preferred drug. Sulfasalazine, especially the generic preparation, is the least expensive 5-ASA drug available (Table 20-2). An explanation of its metabolism, actions, and uses helps one understand the development and application of the newer drugs.

Metabolism

The body's handling of sulfasalazine is complex, yet interesting. The essential features follow. About 20 percent of the drug is absorbed in the small intestine and carried attached to proteins in the blood. It has an affinity for connective tissue, which may explain its efficacy in arthritis. The remaining 80 percent travels to the colon, where intestinal bacteria separate the 5-ASA from its sulfapyridine partner (Figure 20-1). The latter is promptly absorbed into the bloodstream, whereby it is carried to the liver. Here it is metabolized by a process known as acetylation (Figure 20-2).

The 5-ASA is largely excreted in the feces, but some is metabolized by colon epithelial cells. Through a series of experiments conducted in Oxford, it became clear that the therapeutic effect of sulfasalazine is principally, perhaps not exclusively, due to the 5-ASA acting topically on the colon, and that the undesirable effects are largely due to the sulfapyridine.

Why, then, has it taken 50 years for 5-ASA itself to be used in IBD? The answer is that orally administered 5-ASA is absorbed in

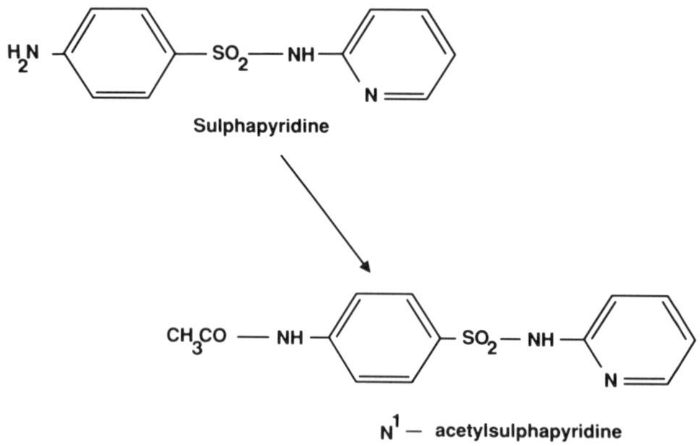

Figure 20-2. The acetylation of sulfapyridine in the liver. Some people are "slow acetylators," who have a reduced tolerance of sulfasalazine.

the small intestine, excreted in the urine, and never reaches the diseased bowel. It thus appears that the 5-ASA acts topically, not via the bloodstream. The pharmaceutical challenge is to devise alternative means by which the drug may be delivered intraluminally to the colon.

Mode of Action

It appears that the sulfapyridine has little therapeutic effect in IBD. It may stop growth of some bacteria, and alter lymphocyte activation, but the importance of these effects is debatable, and attention should be focused on the 5-ASA.

Like its cousin acetylsalicylic acid (aspirin), 5-ASA inhibits two enzymes responsible for the metabolism of arachidonic acid, a lipid substance found attached to cell membranes. These enzymes are cyclooxygenase and lipoxygenase. They release prostaglandins and leukotrienes, which probably play a role in the inflammatory process of ulcerative colitis and Crohn's disease. The 5-ASA has several other possible beneficial actions, such as interference with antibody production, but its exact effects on the inflamed colon mucosa are unknown.

Uses of Sulfasalazine

1. Treatment of mild to moderate ulcerative colitis; in combination with steroids in severe ulcerative colitis; and maintenance therapy for ulcerative colitis in remission (see Chapter 9).
2. Treatment of active colonic Crohn's disease. Because the 5-ASA in sulfasalazine is not released until the drug reaches the colon, and because the action is topical, the drug is not effective in small-bowel Crohn's disease. It appears not to be useful for maintenance of remission of Crohn's, but this is controversial (see Chapter 13).

3. Treatment of rheumatoid arthritis; it may be useful when other drugs fail. Those IBD patients with colitic arthritis or rheumatoid (ankylosing) spondylitis may achieve a double benefit (see Chapter 16).

Unwanted Effects

Sulfasalazine obviously should not be used in people with known sensitivity to sulfonamides or salicylates. Most side-effects are related to the sulfapyridine component of the drug. Among the population there are both rapid and slow acetylators. Because the disposition of sulfapyridine is principally through acetylation in the liver, slow acetylators may metabolize the drug slowly (Figure 20-2). This partly explains why some patients cannot tolerate sulfasalazine in the usual therapeutic doses, but can manage smaller amounts. The list of possible adverse effects of sulfasalazine seems formidable, but most are dose related and reversible if the drug is discontinued. Nevertheless at least 10 percent of people are unable to take this otherwise useful preparation.

Dose-related adverse effects are headaches, nausea, fever, skin rash, itch, dizziness, ringing in the ears, indigestion, swelling about the eyes, and a yellow tint to the skin. An orange tint to the urine may be alarming, but is of no consequence. Often these effects are avoided if the drug is stopped, and restarted at a lower dose. Decreased sperm and infertility may occur in men, but fertility returns when the drug is withdrawn.

More serious but fortunately rare reactions that are independent of dose include hepatitis, hemolytic anemia, kidney failure, various skin eruptions, and lupus erythematosus. Reduced white blood cell count (leukopenia) and platelet count (thrombocytopenia) may be very serious.

A final untoward effect that is not often mentioned is a paradoxical worsening of the IBD. This phenomenon occurs with all the 5-ASA drugs. If a patient's colitis seems to deteriorate on the drug, one should think of this unexpected effect.

Administration

Trade names for sulfasalazine include Salazopyrin and Azulfidine. The drug is available in 500-milligram tablets. The usual maintenance dose for ulcerative colitis is 2 grams a day, taken in divided doses two or four times a day. For active colitis, 8 to 12 tablets a day are recommended (4–6 grams). An even higher dose is sometimes used, but a patient's tolerance for the drug is the limiting factor. Enteric-coated pills are available for those who suffer indigestion with the plain tablets. It is wise to check the white cell and platelet count a week after starting the drug and periodically thereafter. The monthly cost for generic sulfasalazine, 4 grams/day is about $35 Cdn. This is less than half that of the newer 5-ASA preparations (Table 20-2).

OLSALAZINE (DIPENTUM)

If colon bacteria can split the azo bond of sulfasalazine, releasing 5-ASA at its target site of action, why not create a drug consisting of two 5-ASA molecules joined by this same azo bond? Why not indeed, and the result is olsalazine (Figure 20-3). Administered orally, the drug is cleaved by colon bacteria, releasing two 5-ASA molecules. Olsalazine is therefore theoretically as effective as sulfasalazine in the treatment of active colitis, and at half the dose. This is supported by comparison trials. Furthermore, 0.5 gram or 1

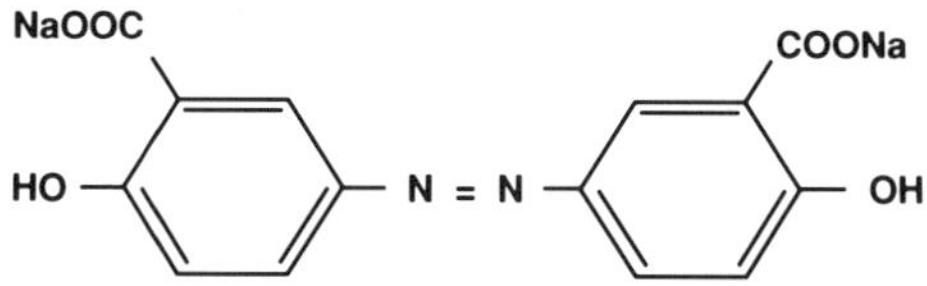

Figure 20-3. Olsalazine. Note the azo bond joining the two 5-ASA molecules. This bond is cleaved by bacteria in the colon in a manner similar to that of sulfasalazine.

gram olsalazine twice daily in two studies appears to be as effective as 1 gram or 2 grams sulfasalazine twice daily in the maintenance of a remission in ulcerative colitis for 48 weeks. Yet another study found that olsalazine was superior to mesalamine in the prevention of relapses of ulcerative colitis. This was especially true for left-sided colitis, perhaps because olsalazine releases 5-ASA farther down the colon than does mesalamine. In the olsalazine/sulfasalazine study, withdrawal from the protocol for side-effects occurred in 7 percent for each drug, but those with previously known side-effects to sulfasalazine had been excluded. As one might expect, olsalazine has no therapeutic effect on arthritis.

However, some side-effects remain. Headache, abdominal pain, nausea, and light-headedness occur. Diarrhea seems to be a common side-effect, but the mechanism is not known. The rare, serious adverse effects that occur with sulfasalazine have not yet been reported, but olsalazine is new, whereas its predecessor has established its reputation over 50 years.

One gram of olsalazine daily (250-milligram capsules four times per day) provides good maintenance of remission in ulcerative colitis. For active ulcerative or Crohn's colitis, 1.5 to 3 grams daily are used. Diarrhea may be a limiting factor in the use of this drug.

MESALAMINE

Asacol

The first and most widely used of the newer 5-ASA preparations, Asacol is embedded in a resin called eudragit S. This substance disintegrates at pH 7, which is close to that pH usually found in the colon. Asacol thus delivers 5-ASA to the colon, where it is released. Most is excreted in the feces. Asacol appears to be as effective as sulfasalazine in the treatment of mild or moderate ulcerative or Crohn's colitis, or the maintenance of remission in ulcerative colitis.

The serious side-effects attributed to the sulfapyridine in sulfasalazine appear to be avoided. Those that do occur are mild and reversible. They include nausea, headache, diarrhea, fever, rash, hair loss, and a paradoxical worsening of the colitis. Low sperm counts and infertility apparently do not occur. For maintenance of remission in ulcerative colitis, one 400-milligram tablet of Asacol is taken three or four times per day. For the treatment of colitis, 2.4 grams or more may be used. Because Asacol has fewer adverse effects than sulfasalazine, larger doses of 5-ASA are permitted. Using 2.4 grams Asacol daily, one study has demonstrated that relapses of Crohn's disease may be reduced, even in ileal disease.

Mesalamine (Salofalk, Claversal, Mesasal)

This preparation is similar to Asacol except that in this case, the resin in which the 5-ASA is imbedded is eudragit L, which disintegrates at pH 6. The pH in the ileum is higher than that in the colon, so 5-ASA is released in the terminal ileum as well as in the colon. Whether or not this preparation is effective in Crohn's disease of the ileum remains to be proven, but it appears to be in widespread use for that purpose. As in the case of Asacol, it seems to be effective for maintenance of remission in ulcerative colitis, although less so than olsalazine. It is also effective in the treatment of active colitis. The unwanted effects are similar to those of Asacol. The 250- and 500-milligram tablets are used in a daily dose similar to that of Asacol.

Mesalamine (Pentasa)

Pentasa is a slow-release mesalamine prepared in microgranules coated with ethylcellulose. The rate of release increases above pH 6, but some discharge occurs independent of pH. Thus, about 60 percent of the ingested drug is made available for topical effect throughout the small bowel. Because only half of this is absorbed, about 70 percent travels to the colon.

Pentasa, therefore, seems well designed to treat small-bowel Crohn's disease, and is already in use for this purpose. Only experience and proper trials will indicate whether or not this policy is justified. Otherwise, the indications and untoward effects are similar to those of the other mesalamines. Tablet strengths are 250 and 500 milligrams.

TOPICAL 5-ASA

Enemas

For patients with proctosigmoiditis or left-sided colitis, a retention enema is an efficient means by which medication can be delivered to the inflamed surface of the colon. Properly applied, an enema can deliver 5-ASA well up the colon, even beyond the splenic flexure.

The available enemas vary from country to country. Salofalk enemas contain 4 grams of 5-ASA in 60 grams of fluid. Expense is a major drawback. Pentasa enemas, available in the United Kingdom, contain 1 gram in 100 grams of fluid, and are designed to release the drug over 6 hours. The greatest benefit can be expected if the enemas are retained for a long period. Sulfasalazine enemas are unavailable in North America, and would seem to offer little advantage over the other two.

In order that the enema be retained along the left colon, one should apply it while lying on the left side, knees drawn up, and with the buttocks supported by a pillow. Before the enema tip is inserted into the anus, it should be lubricated with a water-soluble lubricant or petrolatum (Vaseline). With practice, the enema fluid may be injected up the full length of the left colon, and retained there several hours.

Suppositories

Rectal suppositories containing 5-ASA are useful in ulcerative proctitis, where the medication need be applied only to the distal 8 to 15 centimeters of the colorectum. Salofalk suppositories, 250 or 500 milligrams, are available in North America. The torpedo-shaped suppositories are much easier to manage than enemas, and may be inserted two or three times a day without the need to lie down.

SUMMARY

For 50 years, sulfasalazine has been the standard medication for mild to moderately active ulcerative colitis, and for the maintenance of remission. It appears also to be effective in the treatment of Crohn's colitis, but not disease of the small bowel. Over the years it has become evident that the active component of the drug is the 5-ASA. This salicylate is split from its sulfapyridine partner by bacteria in the colon, where in colitis, it works topically on the inflamed mucosa. The sulfapyridine is held responsible for most of the side-effects of the ingested sulfasalazine. The newer 5-ASA preparations represent attempts to deliver 5-ASA to the site of inflamed bowel without using sulfapyridine. Olsalazine consists of two 5-ASA molecules joined by an azo bond similar to that of sulfasalazine. As in the case of its predecessor, olsalazine is split by colon bacteria releasing, in this case, two 5-ASAs in the colon. In Asacol the salicylate is imbedded in the resin eudragit S, which dissolves in the colon. Other mesalamines employ eudragit L, which releases its load in the ileum and colon. Pentasa is a slow-release mesalamine that distributes 5-ASA throughout the small intestine and colon. These latter two preparations may have some application in small-intestinal Crohn's disease. Large-dose Asacol may be useful for the maintenance of remission in Crohn's. Suppositories or enemas containing 5-ASA are effective in ulcerative proctitis, or proctosigmoiditis. Controlled trials and experience are required to determine the place of these newer salicylate preparations in the management of IBD.

CHAPTER TWENTY-ONE

Steroids

In the 1988 Olympics, the sprinter, Ben Johnson, introduced *steroids* into the popular lexicon. He used anabolic steroids, which (like the male sex hormone, testosterone) increase muscle mass and strength. Clearly, this is *not* the type of steroid that is the subject of this chapter. Steroids are a large group of hormones with profound effects on the body. Sex hormones are steroids, but the term steroids usually refers to hormones secreted by the adrenal gland, or to synthetic drugs such as prednisone, which attempt to maximize therapeutic effects and minimize the unwanted effects of the natural hormones.

The chemical structure of prednisone is illustrated in Figure 21-1. All steroids share the basic ring structure of prednisone, but differ in the structure of the side chains. These different side chains produce radically different effects from steroid to steroid.

FUNCTION

Natural steroid hormones produced by the adrenal gland play a vital role in controlling the body's reaction to stress. They manage such things as the kidney's control of water and salt secretion, and regulate inflammation, blood sugar, and blood pressure. Cortisone and its steroid relatives figure in many diseases. For example, when

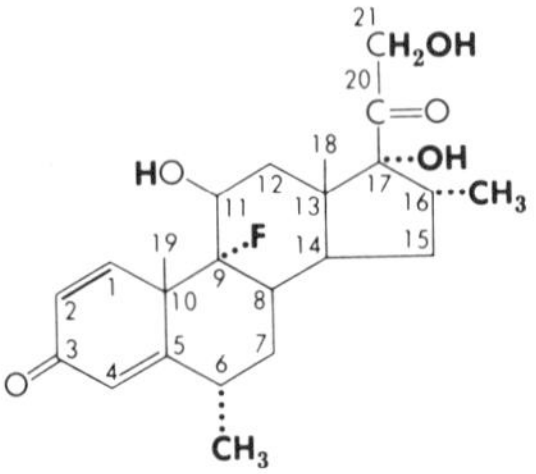

Figure 21-1. Prednisone. Note the four-ring structure, which is common to all steroids. Differences in the side chains account for differences in action.

the adrenal glands are destroyed as in tuberculosis or some cancers, salt loss, low blood sugar, and low blood pressure may result. Potentially fatal, this condition is termed *Addison's disease* and can be treated by certain adrenal steroid drugs.

A similar condition may arise if a patient is suddenly withdrawn from steroids after a prolonged treatment course. The pituitary gland normally stimulates the adrenal glands when steroid is required through the release of adrenocorticotropic hormone (ACTH). Prolonged steroid administration shuts off the pituitary, and the adrenal glands become lazy. When the steroid is withdrawn after prolonged therapy, a hypoadrenalism similar to Addison's disease may result. Subsequently, a sudden stress such as an injury or surgery may increase demand for corticosteroids, and if the adrenal glands cannot respond, substitute steroids must be injected.

Different consequences occur if a tumor of an adrenal gland overproduces steroids. One result is Cushing's syndrome, with salt retention, high blood sugar, and high blood pressure. These and many more *cushingoid* effects are discussed later as side-effects of steroid treatment.

USES OF STEROIDS

There are many conditions of which we do not know the cause. Some, such as ulcerative colitis, Crohn's disease, and chronic active hepatitis, are inflammatory conditions. These are believed by some to be due to a disorder, or perhaps an overactivity, of the immune system. Steroids are used because of their effects in suppressing inflammation and altering the body's immune response. Their antiinflammatory effects are useful in many medical conditions in which *autoimmunity* is believed to be active. Like 5-aminosalicylic acid, steroids may also act in part by suppressing production of prostaglandins and leukotrienes.

The use of cortisone in the treatment of ulcerative colitis was first validated by Truelove and Witts in 1955. These authors compared 150 milligrams of cortisone with placebo in 197 British patients. This is a small dose by today's standards (equal to prednisone, 20 milligrams/day). These same authors proved that the adrenal-stimulating pituitary hormone ACTH is as effective, but it is seldom employed now. Another British group showed that a maintenance dose of 15 milligrams prednisone per day was no better than placebo in preventing relapses. For the proof that prednisone is effective in Crohn's disease, we turn to the United States and European Cooperative Crohn's Disease studies (Chapter 24).

Steroids are the most effective agents we have for the management of active ulcerative colitis and Crohn's disease. Other drugs have a supportive role in certain circumstances, and occasionally a mild colitis may be treated with sulfasalazine or 5-aminosalicylic acid (5-ASA, mesalamine). Most patients, however, will need steroids at some point. Clinical trials support the use of steroids in severe ulcerative colitis and Crohn's disease. No other drug or method of treatment is as reliable, although there are small studies suggesting efficacy of 6-mercaptopurine (6-MP) or an elemental diet in Crohn's disease.

METHOD OF ADMINISTRATION

Steroid drugs have complex effects and must be taken only with the close guidance of a physician skilled in their use for these diseases. The physician is guided by three principles:

1. Because the benefits of the drug appear to be antiinflammatory, they should be employed only when inflammation is active.

2. Because the undesirable affects are usually related to dose and duration of administration, they should be reduced once the inflammation is under control.

3. Because all steroids, even when given topically as a suppository or enema, may suppress the adrenal gland, and because steroids suppress rather than extinguish inflammation, they should never be stopped abruptly. Rather, they should be tapered slowly in 5- or 2.5-milligram decrements at 5- to 7-day intervals until the dose becomes zero. If signs of inflammation intervene, a period of stable therapy at the minimal effective dose is usually indicated. A few weeks later, one should again attempt to taper the dose.

Prednisone is a tablet usually of 5-milligram strength. Because this synthetic steroid minimizes some of the undesirable effects of the natural hormone and has been well studied in the therapy of inflammatory bowel disease (IBD), it is the most common oral form used. There are also steroid enemas (hydrocortisone, betamethasone) and suppositories (hydrocortisone) for local therapy of the rectum and lower colon. Intravenous steroids (hydrocortisone, methylprednisolone) are used in severe acute attacks when oral administration is not possible or desirable.

UNDESIRABLE EFFECTS

Because steroids, even synthetic ones, have profound effects on every cell of the body, consequences other than the desired therapeutic ones can be expected. Most patients can tolerate prednisone safely in high doses for short periods. However, large doses over a long time carry an increasing risk of side-effects. This is the reason that the high dose used for the management of acute attacks should be promptly reduced as the inflammation is suppressed. There is a great deal of individual variation, however, both in the occurrence of these undesirable effects and in the dose needed to suppress the disease. In most individuals the drug is tolerated well, and the benefits in terms of control of the disease far outweigh the risks. Nonetheless, one should be aware of the following possible side-effects. This list is not complete, and some putative side-effects, such as peptic ulcer, are debatable.

Cosmetic and Psychological Effects

Most people taking steroids feel an increase in appetite, and this, along with fluid retention, may lead to weight gain. Stretch marks may occur in the skin, particularly in the abdomen. The skin is thinned, and bruising is common. Some women may develop facial hair. Young people may develop acne, and in some cases, this requires dermatologic care. The face may be rounded, and in some, a "buffalo hump" appears high in the back.

Some individuals experience a change in mood that may range from depression through irritability to elation. Reduction in the dose and eventual cessation of the drug will reverse most of these phenomena.

Metabolic Effects

Potentially more serious adverse effects include an elevation of the blood pressure and worsening or unmasking of diabetes. In postmenopausal women there is an increased risk of osteoporosis (i.e., weakening of the bones); thus, fractures can be a consequence of long-term steroids. The disease that is being treated, of course, may participate in some of these adverse effects as well. Rarely there may be interference with the blood supply to the hip, leading to damage severe enough to require orthopedic surgery (aseptic necrosis of the hip). This usually requires an artificial joint. Increased pressure in the eye may occur, and cataracts are more common in those who have taken long-term steroids.

Altered Resistance to Infection

Steroids may interfere with the body's ability to defend itself; thus, the inflammatory and immune reaction to infections may be impaired. For example, tuberculosis may become active in patients who already harbor the disease. Bacterial infections may be more severe than normal. Healing following surgery may also be impaired. In seriously ill patients, steroids may suppress the usual physical signs that warn of abscess or perforation, and dangerously delay surgery.

Adrenal Suppression

As mentioned previously, long-standing treatment with prednisone may suppress the adrenal glands' ability to secrete natural hormones. Those who have been on steroids for a long time should carry this information on their persons. A "medi-alert" bracelet is suitable for this purpose. In the case of an accident or emergency surgery, these hormones may need to be administered intravenously to mimic the adrenal glands' normal response to stress.

Steroid Dependency

It must be stressed that the serious reactions mentioned are rare if large doses of the drug are confined to brief periods, and the patient is quickly tapered off the drug or maintained for short periods on the minimal dose necessary to control the disease. There is unfortunately no satisfactory substitute for prednisone in severe disease. The benefits of steroid therapy are often very satisfying, especially when treatment is tailored to each patient's need and carefully monitored by a physician.

After many months of steroid therapy, during which there have been several unsuccessful attempts by the patient to wean him- or herself off the drug, he or she is said to be steroid dependent. Especially if side-effects are severe, alternatives should be sought. Surgery may be indicated, especially where cure is possible, as in ulcerative colitis. Sometimes, in Crohn's disease, there has been previous surgery with recurrent disease. In this situation further surgery may not be an option, and azathioprine or 6-MP may be justified (Chapter 22). These toxic immunosuppressants at least reduce steroid need, and at most may permit their complete withdrawal.

TOPICAL STEROIDS

Topical steroid enemas or suppositories have been used with success in proctosigmoiditis or proctitis. In theory, enemas and suppositories deliver a maximal amount of drug to the inflamed area, with minimal side-effects. Some steroid is absorbed, however, perhaps more when the area is inflamed, and it is not rare to observe cushingoid effects in patients using these rectal preparations.

Dexamethasone or hydrocortisone rectal enemas are available, and are administered in the manner described for 5-ASA enemas (see Chapter 20). Hydrocortisone acetate (Cortifoam) is a popular variation on this theme. Steroid suppositories, unencumbered with other drugs, are not so readily available. Hydrocortisone acetate (Cortament) suppositories are useful in 10- and 40-milligram doses for ulcerative proctitis.

FUTURE CONSIDERATIONS

A drug that combines the beneficial effects of steroids in IBD with no untoward effects would revolutionize the management of these disorders. Several new developments may make such a remedy possible. New steroid topical preparations have been developed that are potent, yet because they are not absorbed or quickly destroyed in the liver, they have minimal side-effects. These drugs, beclomethasone dipropionate and budesonide, have been proposed as per anal treatment of ulcerative colitis, and the latter, for oral treatment of ileocecal Crohn's disease. Clinical trials are in progress.

SUMMARY

There are many steroid hormones, each with profound physiologic effects. In relation to IBD, steroid refers to adrenocortical hormones produced by the adrenal glands under pituitary control. Synthetic adrenal steroids, such as oral prednisone, intravenous methylprednisolone, or topical betamethasone, have been used therapeutically because they have less severe untoward effects than do their natural cousins. These drugs are effective in IBD because they have antiimmune and antiinflammatory effects, but their precise mode of action is a mystery. Unfortunately, they have undesirable side-effects, which may be cosmetic or metabolic, or may depress the body's reaction to infection or stress. These drugs thus should be used only when the IBD is active, in the minimal effective dose, for the shortest possible period. To this end, once remission is achieved, an initial daily dose of 40 to 60 milligrams of prednisone is tapered step-wise at 5- to 7-day intervals until the patient is either off the drug, or the lowest effective dose has been reached. Because of adrenal suppression, the drug should never be abruptly stopped, yet chronic use should be avoided by periodic attempts to further taper the dose.

CHAPTER TWENTY-TWO
Immunosuppressives

Primum, non nocere [First, do no harm].
Anonymous

Immunosuppressive drugs suppress the cellular components of the immune system. Because disordered immunity is believed by many to execute the gut damage seen in inflammatory bowel disease (IBD), it is reasoned that immune suppression could be beneficial. Some clinical trials support this reasoning. Unfortunately immuno-suppressant drugs suppress other cells as well, notably those of the bone marrow. The resulting decrease in white cells or platelets in the blood could permit uncontrolled infection or bleeding. Furthermore, the immune system itself is there for a purpose. The cellular components of immunity seek and destroy foreign substances or antigens, such as microorganisms or cancer cells, capable of harm. Moreover, some of these drugs are known to cause cancer in some situations, and there is concern about possible effects on repro-duction. For these reasons their use is very controversial. The growing realization that immunosuppressives have a place in the therapy of Crohn's disease is tempered by the fear of devastating adverse effects on the very young people who are most likely to benefit. Of course, steroids and the disease itself are not without harm; therefore, the use of these sometimes toxic drugs is a judgment call that depends on circumstances, and requires the utmost understanding and cooperation of the patient.

AZATHIOPRINE (IMURAN)

This drug was used to prevent rejection of human organ transplants, but now is largely supplanted by cyclosporine for this purpose. Azathioprine is also used in several medical disorders believed due to a deranged immune system. These include chronic active hepatitis, severe rheumatoid arthritis, lupus erythematosus, polyarteritis nodosa, and pemphigus. It is seldom considered a first-line drug for any of these conditions, nor should it be for Crohn's disease.

Many of the actions of this drug are attributable to its principal metabolite, 6-mercaptopurine (6-MP). In IBD, the two drugs are often considered interchangeable. Double-blind trials of azathioprine in Crohn's disease have tended to be either very small or not convincing. A British study showed a small, statistically insignificant benefit, but the authors offered qualified support for its use in some patients. The National Cooperative Crohn's Disease Study (NCCDS) found that azathioprine alone was of no benefit, but that it often permitted a reduction in the dose of prednisone. Critics note that the NCCDS used a very small dose of the drug, and that the 17-week duration of the trial may have been insufficient for the drug to take effect. 6-Mercaptopurine tends to be used more often than azathioprine for the treatment of Crohn's disease, and a positive trial using this drug will be discussed.

The commonest adverse effects of azathioprine occur as a result of bone marrow suppression. Regular white blood cell and platelet counts are therefore necessary when taking this drug, lest severe leukopenia occur, with impaired resistance to infection, or thrombocytopenia low platelets with bleeding. Liver damage, pancreatitis, and skin eruptions are other potential adverse reactions. When employed as an antirejection drug for kidney transplant patients, azathioprine has apparently caused cancer in a few cases. This fear of cancer at some future date and the unknown effects on unborn children inspire caution in the use of this drug, especially in the case of children and women of childbearing age.

The drug is available in 25-milligram tablets, and a common starting dose is 50 milligrams per day. While monitoring the white cell count weekly, the dose may be increased to 1 to 2 milligrams/kilogram body weight per day. Generally a smaller dose is required than that for transplant patients.

6-MERCAPTOPURINE (MERCAPTAN)

As mentioned, 6-MP is a metabolic product of azathioprine, and data from the study of either drug are often, perhaps unjustifiably, used interchangeably. 6-Mercaptopurine, however, is most commonly used in the treatment of certain types of leukemia, whereas azathioprine has a role in organ transplantation. The comparative dose of 6-MP is 55 percent that of azathioprine.

The use of 6-MP in Crohn's disease is based largely on a controlled trial conducted by gastroenterologists at the Mt. Sinai Hospital, New York, in 1980. Although much clinical experience has accumulated since that time, no other controlled studies have been forthcoming. The same group also demonstrated that Crohn's fistulas closed in most of their patients taking 6-MP, but an average of 3 months was required. The fistulas recurred if the drug was withdrawn.

Most gastroenterologists agree that 6-MP has a place in the management of Crohn's disease, but differ as to what that place should be. Although some are enthusiastic about this drug, and even consider it a first-line therapy for Crohn's disease, most physicians are very hesitant to employ it. This is because of its uncommon, but severe, short-term, adverse effects and unknown long-term consequences. In the Mt. Sinai study, the drug had to be withdrawn in 10 percent of cases. The 3 months' wait for beneficial effects is a disadvantage for the severely ill patient for whom a decision to operate hangs in the balance.

Leukopenia (low white blood cell count) is a major risk. The white count should be closely monitored, especially as the drug is introduced. The total white cell count is less important than the neutrophil (polymorph) count. Deficient polymorphs impair the body's ability to resist acute infections, and the consequences can be very serious. This marrow suppression may be enhanced if the drug allopurinol (used for gout) is given with 6-MP.

Jaundice, stomatitis (mouth sores), nausea, vomiting, and lung infiltration rarely occur, but the most feared short-term complication is pancreatitis. Among nearly 400 patients taking 6-MP for an average of 5 years, pancreatitis occurred in 3.3 percent; bone marrow depression, in 2 percent; allergic reactions, in 2 percent; and infections, some life threatening, in 7 percent. Advocates of 6-MP rightly point out that prednisone has serious adverse effects as well, but it is the possible future development of cancer or alteration in reproductive cells that causes most physicians to hesitate to recommend this drug. Most would reserve it for those patients with Crohn's disease who fail to respond to adequate doses of prednisone, or who are steroid dependent, and in whom surgery is not a viable option. Such a situation might arise when the patient has already had surgical procedures, or when he or she refuses an operation. The drug may have a place in the healing of fistulas, but again, the 3-month lag period and risk of superinfection make it unattractive. In my opinion, there is little evidence to support the use of 6-MP in ulcerative colitis. When steroid resistance or dependency occurs, colectomy seems a better option.

For Crohn's disease, 50-milligram tablets of 6-MP are given daily, and the white count is estimated first weekly, and then twice monthly. The dose may be cautiously increased to 75 or rarely 100 milligrams over several weeks. The maximum dose is approximately 1.1 milligram/kilogram body weight per day. Once the drug is established, other drugs, notably prednisone, should be cautiously withdrawn. The drug may be required for years, and withdrawal may be accompanied by disease recurrence. Concomitant administration of folinic acid, or folic acid (which is cheaper), may prevent marrow suppression. If pregnancy is contemplated, the drug must be discontinued (see Chapter 19).

METHOTREXATE

Methotrexate is an antimetabolic, anti-inflammatory, and folic acid antagonist drug with immune-suppressing effect. It is used in the chemotherapy of some cancers, and increasingly in the treatment of some chronic inflammatory disorders in which disordered immunity is deemed important. Examples are psoriasis and rheumatoid arthritis. A small, uncontrolled trial suggests a role for this drug in IBD, and controlled studies are urgently needed to confirm this. Our desperate need for effective therapy for chronic active Crohn's disease should not permit this drug's general use without better proof of efficacy. Methotrexate, therefore, should not yet be administered for Crohn's disease outside clinical trials.

The drug is given in weekly intramuscular injections of 15 to 25 milligrams. This avoids the nausea that accompanies oral administration, and accumulation of the drug, which occurs with daily dosing. Methotrexate has definite effects on the fetus, so adequate birth control is essential. Abortion may occur if the drug is given in pregnancy. Liver toxicity is common in patients receiving the drug, and may prove to be a deterrent to its use in IBD. The weekly dosing may minimize liver damage. Marrow suppression, mouth ulcers, and kidney damage are other adverse effects of this drug.

CYCLOSPORIN A

Cyclosporine (cyclosporin A) has revolutionized organ transplantation. Small open trials suggest a role for this drug in Crohn's disease, as they have for methotrexate. A small, flawed, controlled trial suggests efficacy, but more studies are required before the drug should be used generally for the treatment of Crohn's disease.

A multicentered, controlled Canadian trial demonstrates that cyclosporine in small doses (average 4.8 milligram/day) is not only of no benefit in the maintenance of remission from Crohn's disease, but also that it may actually do harm. This serves as a timely reminder of the need for such studies for all IBD treatments. This very important concept is pursued further in Chapter 24.

Cyclosporine is toxic to the kidney, and the dose should be closely monitored by serial cyclosporine blood levels. Tremors, convulsions, and high blood pressure are other untoward effects.

SUMMARY

The decision to use immunosuppressives in Crohn's disease requires careful assessment of the severity of the disease, the adverse effects of the drug, the patient's understanding of these effects, and his or her willingness to cooperate with the monitoring process. They are not first-line drugs in the treatment of Crohn's disease, and careful analysis of the data suggests that their overall efficacy is not great. The short-term risk of untoward effects, such as pancreatitis or marrow suppression, may be acceptable in severe, intractable disease, but the unknown risk of future cancers or birth defects is troubling. Perhaps 6-MP is the immunosuppressive to choose at this time, although others eventually may prove to be better. Despite enthusiasm by some, a safe, conservative position is that these toxic drugs should be reserved for those patients with steroid-resistant, or steroid-dependent Crohn's disease, in which surgery is not an option. Because surgery is curative, there seems to be no place for immunosuppressives in ulcerative colitis.

CHAPTER TWENTY-THREE
Antibiotics

Most antibiotics have no effect on uncomplicated inflammatory bowel disease (IBD). Nevertheless, septic complications are common in Crohn's disease, because of its tendency to create fistulas and abscesses. These infections often require more than one antibiotic in order to cope with the diverse organisms originating in the gut. Broad-spectrum antibiotics such as tetracycline are sometimes used in Crohn's disease to suppress bacteria that may be abnormally present in the small intestine, where they impair nutrient absorption (see Chapter 14). In fulminant colitis or an attack of Crohn's disease with high fever, antibiotics are sometimes used to minimize the risk of septic complications (see Chapter 10). Beyond these applications, antibiotics do not attack Crohn's disease itself. There is one exception. Metronidazole benefits patients with Crohn's colitis or perianal disease, apparently through something other than its antibacterial effect.

METRONIDAZOLE (FLAGYL)

Metronidazole has many antimicrobial uses. It is effective against several parasitic protozoan infections, such as trichomonas in the vagina, giardia in the small intestine, and ameba in the colon.

The drug is also effective against many bacteria resident in the colon, especially the predominant anaerobes (bacteria that grow in the absence of air). Because of this feature, metronidazole is commonly used as a bowel preparation before intestinal surgery, and for infections generated by fecal organisms. It also accounts for its use for the septic complications of Crohn's disease. Another important indication for the drug is antibiotic-associated (pseudomembranous) colitis, in which the offending organism is the toxin-producing *Clostridium difficile*.

Clinical Data

Metronidazole merits special mention here because of its unique benefit to patients with Crohn's colitis or perianal fistulas. One controlled study in Sweden demonstrated that this drug is at least as effective as sulfasalazine in Crohn's disease of the colon. Furthermore, those who did not improve on sulfasalazine did so when switched to metronidazole, whereas the reverse was not true. Uncontrolled studies show impressive results when this drug is used for perianal fistulas. Although controlled studies would be more credible, they would be very difficult to perform in this case. The drug must be carefully withdrawn, as relapses are common. Sometimes therapy must be continued for many months or years.

A North American trial compared two doses of metronidazole 20 milligrams/kilogram/day and 10 milligrams/kilogram/day with placebo in the treatment of acute attacks of Crohn's disease. The study is flawed in that only 56 of 105 patients completed the course of treatment. The larger dose seemed more effective than the smaller one, but neither was significantly better than placebo. Only when the two treated groups were lumped together did the drug appear to have a statistically beneficial effect.

The mechanism of metronidazole's action in Crohn's disease is unknown. It may yet prove to be the drug's antibacterial action, especially against the anaerobic bacteroides species, that permits healing. If this were the case, however, antibiotics with similar activity should work, and they don't. Metronidazole apparently suppresses cell-mediated immunity, but the importance of this is unknown.

Precautions and Adverse Effects

The most serious adverse effects of this drug are neurological. Seizures and sensory peripheral nerve deficits occur rarely at the low doses commonly employed for Crohn's disease. The drug interferes with the metabolism of alcohol in a manner similar to that of disulfiram (antabuse). The latter is sometimes used to decondition alcoholics to alcohol, producing a violent reaction when the two are taken together. Thus metronidazole treatment imposes abstinence, not in itself a bad thing! A prolonged high dose may depress the white blood cell count. The commonest reactions, though, are nausea, vomiting, abdominal pain, loss of appetite, and a metallic taste. Skin rashes are rare. The urine may become dark reddish brown, which can be alarming if the patient is not forewarned. A fungal infection of the vagina may occur, as the normal local bacterial flora is suppressed.

Metronidazole thus has a limited place in the treatment of Crohn's colitis, especially if the 5-aminosalicylic acid (5-ASA) compounds cannot be used. It may assist the healing of perianal fistulas, and avoid or reduce the necessity for steroids. There seems to be no support for its use in small-bowel disease or in ulcerative colitis. Even for Crohn's colitis, it is a second or third choice. It must be given with caution in the presence of liver or kidney disease.

Administration

The Swedish trial employed 0.8 gram of metronidazole per day, but twice that dose is often used. In the North American study 10 and 20 milligrams/kilogram body weight were used, which, for a 50-kilogram or 120-pound person works out to 500 milligrams or 1 gram/day. There are many tablet strengths: 250, 400, and 500 milligrams, and the drug is also available as an intravenous preparation. A common regimen is 500 milligrams, two or three times per day.

SUMMARY

Although several antibiotics are needed for the various septic complications of Crohn's disease, only metronidazole appears to have a therapeutic effect on the disease itself. It is at least as useful as sulfasalazine in the treatment of Crohn's colitis, and may aid the healing of perianal fistulas. The side-effects are significant, and the drug is used only when others are not effective.

CHAPTER TWENTY-FOUR

Placebos and Clinical Trials

Mark Twain once facetiously remarked that it takes less moral courage to administer a pill than it does to swallow it. However untrue this may be, patients deserve reassurance that the drugs they employ are effective and safe. Inflammatory bowel disease (IBD) features relapses and remissions. Every patient receives some treatment, but how can we be sure that remission would not have occurred without treatment? Indeed, might not the patient be better off without treatment? Clinical trials attempt to answer these questions in a rational, scientific manner, but trials in IBD are very complicated. Here we discuss the need for and the principles of clinical trials, how benefit might be measured, and the obscure, even mystical effects of placebos.

NEED FOR TRIALS IN IBD

When a surgeon lances a boil, relief is instantaneous. Science is observation, and no one doubts the efficacy of this procedure. Penicillin in pneumococcal pneumonia or colectomy for toxic mega-colon are readily seen to be effective, even life-saving. In these cases the illness is acute, the treatment is specific, and the end-point (cure) is obvious. In a chronic, fluctuating disease such as ulcerative colitis or Crohn's disease, however, most medical and surgical treatments are not so easy to validate. Much of therapeutics is instinctive and sensible, but lacks proof of efficacy.

Treatment efficacy is difficult to establish when a measurable end-point such as cure or improvement is neither rapid nor obvious. Observations of the chronic, fluctuating symptoms and signs of IBD should be objective; that is, improvement or lack of it should be recognizable by other than the doctor and the patient, whose biases may cloud their judgment. In IBD, the activity of the disease is difficult to judge and, despite some objective tests and signs, the symptoms are subjective and the changes, subtle. It may take some weeks or months before improvement may be registered. The IBD patient is seldom cured, so judgment of improvement is subject to many biases resulting from individual interpretation, changing attitudes, hope, and what is known as the placebo response (see the following). To circumvent these biases, the clinical trial has been developed. This technique is now commonplace and is responsible for the validation of many treatments employed in IBD.

PRINCIPLES OF A CLINICAL TRIAL

The simplest clinical trial is that carried out daily in the doctor's office. For a patient's symptom, the doctor tries a drug or diet based on his or her experience and knowledge. If the symptom is improved with no harmful side-effect, all is well. Often the doctor cannot prove from the available published literature that the treatment is generally effective for that symptom. If he or she finds that the treatment satisfies most patients with similar symptoms, the doctor gains confidence with it and uses it again, sometimes for other symptoms as well. This process, however pragmatic and sensible, is quite unscientific and subject to bias. How else might one explain why blood-letting, acupuncture, megavitamins, and environmental treatments became so fashionable in their times?

Recognition of bias led to the concept of the controlled clinical trial. The first such trial was undertaken by James Lind, a British naval surgeon on board the H.M.S. Salisbury in 1747. Contemporary sailors suffered and died of scurvy during long sea voyages. We now know that this was due to the dietary lack of vitamin C–containing fruits and vegetables. Many noxious nostrums were employed as treatment of this disease without scientific validation, and certainly without success. In order to discredit the nostrums and convince naval authorities of the value of fruits, Lind conducted the following clinical trial.

> On the 20th of May 1747, I took 12 patients in the scurvy on board the Salisbury at sea. Their cases were as similar as I could have them. They all in general had putrid gums, the spots and lassitude, with weakness of their knees. They lay together in one place, being a proper apartment for the sick in the forehold; and one diet common to all. . . . Two of these were ordered each a quart of cider a day. Two others took 25 gutts of elixir vitriol 3 times a day. . . . Two others took 2 teaspoons of vinegar 3 times a day. . . . Two . . . were put on a course of sea water . . . two others had each 2 oranges and one lemon given them every day. . . . The two remaining patients took the bigness of a nutmeg 3 times a day, of an electuary recommended by a hospital surgeon, made of garlic, mustard seed, . . . balsam of Peru, and gum myrrh using a common drink, barley water well assimilated with tamarinds; by a decoction of which, with the addition of cream of tartar, they were gently purged 3 or 4 times during the course. The consequence was that the most sudden and visible good effects were perceived from the use of oranges and lemons; one of those who had taken them being at the end of 6 days fit for duty.

Lind's work led to the virtual eradication of scurvy at sea. British sailors became known as "limeys" because of their daily ration of citrus fruit. Note that the patients all had similar disease, surroundings, and diet; only the treatment varied among the six pairs. With several refinements, such controlled clinical trials are in common use today in all fields of medicine. Treatments are now usually blinded, so that the patient does not know which treatment he is receiving and therefore cannot bias the results. This blinding is usually achieved through the use of a placebo pill that is outwardly identical to the drug under study. The research physician is also biased. His enthusiasm for a new treatment must be controlled, so studies become double-blinded; that is, only a third party knows which treatment the subject receives. An observer's assessment of improvement is therefore free of bias.

The randomized, double-blind, placebo-controlled clinical trial is a vital instrument to validate the efficacy of treatments new and old. Before we consider clinical trials in IBD, we must understand placebos.

PLACEBOS

The efficient physician is the man who successfully amuses his patients while Nature effects a cure.

Voltaire (1694–1778)

It is clear that the placebo response is much more complex than was originally thought, and that it plays a role in almost every therapeutic encounter. Whenever supposedly inert material is given in experimental therapy, as many as half the recipients seem to benefit. For an in-depth discussion of the nature and ethics of placebos, please refer to the article by Brody.

Derived from Latin, *placebo* means *I shall please*. Sugar pills or other harmless remedies have long been employed by physicians. They seemed to work, and patients seemed unhappy if they were given nothing. Because the need to take something is so deeply ingrained in our culture, one might reason that if they work, why not use them? Some, however, express ethical concerns raised by the deception and paternalism implied by this device. It is now appreciated that placebos have measurable effects that may be achieved without deception.

When placebos are given for pain, narcoticlike substances called endorphins, which have pain-relieving qualities, are released in the tissues. The pain relief by placebos may be inhibited by naloxone, a morphine antagonist. Furthermore, in clinical trials, patients warned of possible side-effects of the active drug report experiencing them on the placebo. In fact in several Crohn's disease treatment trials, 6 to 8 percent of patients receiving the inert medication experienced side-effects, forcing withdrawal from the trial. Some people even develop addiction to placebos. Clearly, mind–gut interaction is important in the placebo response. We should recognize that the placebo phenomenon affects every therapeutic interaction. Any medicine works better when given by a caring physician. Surgical removal of a normal organ may have a happy result. It is held by some that even psychotherapy is an elaborate, and expensive, placebo. In the therapy of IBD, and in the interpretation of clinical trials, the placebo effect must be kept clearly in focus.

Placebos and the Natural History of IBD

Since ulcerative colitis and Crohn's disease were recognized early in this century, almost every diagnosed case has received some treatment; therefore, it is difficult to determine the natural history of these diseases. We sense a vast improvement in patients' well-being with modern treatment methods, but we do not know exactly how well they would have done if no treatment had been given. One might learn something of this by studying the fate of those receiving placebos in the published treatment trials of IBD. This is not entirely satisfactory, however, because we know that placebos themselves have some therapeutic effect. Even the placebo recipients receive nutritional and emotional support and careful attention to individual symptoms. Furthermore, trial participants receive placebos for at most 2 years, a brief moment in the long-term course of IBD.

Meyers and Janowitz have reviewed the effect of placebos in Crohn's disease, notably in the large National and European Cooperative Crohn's Disease studies. Here, 178 and 110 patients, respectively, received placebos. They concluded that over a 4-month period, between 25 and 40 percent of patients receiving placebos achieved remission. About 20 percent remained well at 1 year, and 10 percent, at 2 years. If a remission occurred early in the study, there was an improved likelihood that it would be maintained. When another group of patients who were already in remission were studied, 75 percent of those on placebo were in remission at 1 year, and 63 percent, at 2 years. Clearly, any drug proposed for the treatment of this disease, especially if costly or toxic, must be shown to improve these figures. The need for clinical trials that compare the putative therapeutic agent with a placebo is obvious.

Measuring Disease Activity

Clinical trials are relatively easy to perform in ulcerative colitis. The presentation of the disease is fairly uniform and confined to the colon. Progress may be regularly and objectively assessed by sigmoidoscopic examination. As a result, the roles of sulfasalazine and corticosteroids in the treatment and remission-maintenance of ulcerative colitis were established many years ago.

Validation of drug therapy has proven much more difficult in Crohn's disease, in which the manifestations are protean, several levels of the gut may be affected, and often the diseased area is not readily observed. Early treatment was extrapolated uncritically from the experience with ulcerative colitis. Measurement of disease severity and progress in Crohn's disease is often indirect, depending on laboratory tests, body temperature, and the patient's interpretation of symptoms. A further restriction in clinical trials is the need to select patients who are ill enough to require some treatment, yet not so ill that they cannot be observed for a long period, possibly on placebo, as ambulatory patients. Because of these complexities, there are seldom sufficient patients in a single practice or health science center to constitute a valid clinical trial. This is especially so if several drugs are to be tested, and distinction is to be made between various disease presentations.

Hence multicenter trials have become the norm. In the National Cooperative Crohn's Disease Study, for example, 14 United States centers entered a total of 604 patients for the study of three drugs in large- and small-bowel disease over 2 years. Such a large study involves many observers, and therefore requires standardization and a common language. All must agree on the activity of a given case before, throughout, and after treatment. Such a language is the Crohn's Disease Activity Index (CDAI), developed expressly for this study. It has been used in various modified forms in almost every subsequent clinical trial.

The CDAI is summarized in Table 24-1. By this means the symptoms and physical and laboratory manifestations of Crohn's disease are recorded and assigned a weight. The CDAI may be administered in a standardized manner by a trained physician or nurse. Although state of the art, this index has several shortcomings. It does not measure the actual inflammatory activity, nor does it take into account the effect of disease and treatment on quality of life (see Chapter 18). Nevertheless, as the only act in town, some version of this index will be a part of clinical trials in Crohn's disease for the foreseeable future.

TABLE 24-1
Crohn's Disease Activity Index[a]

(× 2) 1.	Number of liquid or very soft stools in one week.
(× 5) 2.	Sum of 7 daily pain ratings: 0 = none; 1 = mild; 2 = moderate; 3 = severe.
(× 7) 3.	Sum of daily ratings of general well-being: 0 = generally well; 1 = slightly below par; 2 = poor; 3 = very poor.
(× 20) 4.	Symptoms or findings presumed related to Crohn's disease a. Arthritis/arthralgia b. Skin/mouth lesions, pyoderma gangrenosa/erythema nodosum c. Iritis/uveitis d. Anal fissure, fistula, or perirectal abscess e. Other bowel-related fistula (e.g., enterovesicle) f. Fever over 37.8°C, or 100°F
(× 30) 5.	Use of diphenoxylate, loperamide, or other opiate for diarrhea: 0 = no, 1 = yes.
(× 10) 6.	Abdominal mass: 0 = absence; 0.4 = questionable; 1 = present.
(× 6) 7.	47 minus hematocrit (males); 42 minus hematocrit (females)
(× 1) 8.	100 × [minus (body weight/standard weight)]

[a]These eight criteria compromise the CDAI. Weighting for each item is indicated in brackets.

TABLE 24-2
Clinical Trials in Ulcerative Colitis

Author	Number of patients	Drug(s)	Time	Study type	Results
Truelove & Witts, 1955	210	Cortisone	6 wk	Active treatment	Doses up to 100 mg/day effective (equiv 20 mg prednisone)
Truelove & Witts, 1959	169	Cortisone vs corticotropin (ACTH)	6 wk	Active treatment	Corticotropin 80 U better than cortisone "little to choose"
Kaplan et al, 1975	22	Hydrocortisone vs ACTH	5–10 days	Active treatment	No difference
Meyers et al, 1983	66	Hydrocortisone vs ACTH	10 days	Active treatment	ACTH better for first attack
Jewell & Truelove, 1974	80	Azathioprine	1 yr	Active treatment	No benefit Maintenance useful in steroid failure
Svartz, 1948	124	Sulfasalazine		Active treatment	First effective therapy
Baron, 1962	50	Sulfasalazine	3 wk	Active treatment	Useful for mild attack of UC

Study					Results
Lennard-Jones et al, 1960	97	Sulfasalazine, prednisone, hydrocortisone enemas	3 wk	Active treatment	Sulfasalazine almost as effective as prednisone. Hydrocortisone enemas less effective in extensive disease
Lennard-Jones et al, 1965	67	Sulfasalazine	1 yr	Maintenance	Reduced attacks
Dissanayake & Truelove, 1973	64	Sulfasalazine	6 mo	Maintenance	2 grams/day effective prophylaxis against recurrence
Riley et al, 1988	88	Sulfasalazine, mesalamine (Asacol)	48 wk	Maintenance	Equivalent doses: 1 gram sulfasalazine = 400 mg mesalamine; no difference in relapses; fewer side effects with mesalamine
Rijk et al, 1992	46	Sulfasalazine, olsalazine	48 wk	Maintenance	Olsalazine, 2 grams/day is as effective as sulfasalazine 4 grams/day
Riley et al, 1988	88	Sulfasalazine, mesalamine (Asacol)	48 wk	Maintenance	Equivalent doses: 1 gram sulfasalazine = 400 mg mesalamine; no difference in relapses; fewer side effects with mesalamine
Courtney et al, 1992	100	Olsalazine, mesalamine	1 yr	Maintenance	Olsalazine, 1 gram/day superior to mesalamine 1.2 gram/day, especially distal colitis

TABLE 24-3
Clinical Trials in Crohn's Disease

Author	Number of patients	Drug(s)	Time	Study type	Results
Summers et al, NCCDS, 1979	569	Prednisone, azathioprine, sulfasalazine	4 mo	Active treatment	Prednisone effective esp. in small bowel; azathioprine not effective, but steroid-sparing; sulfasalazine effective in colon
		Sulfasalazine		Maintenance	Sulfasalazine not effective
Malchow et al, ECCDS, 1984	542	6-Methylprednisolone, sulfasalazine, combination, and placebo	6 mo	Active disease	6-Methylprednisolone best overall. Combo useful in untreated cases and colon
				Maintenance	No value
Singleton et al, NCCDS, 1979	89	Sulfasalazine + prednisone vs. prednisone alone	8 wk	Active treatment	Combination less effective than prednisone alone; no steroid sparing
Rijk et al, 1991	60	Sulfasalazine and prednisone vs prednisone alone	16 wk	Treatment	Prednisone 30 mg/day plus sulfasalazine 6 gm/day induces faster remission than sulfasalazine alone, but same at 16 weeks

Present *et al*, 1980	83	6-Mercaptopurine	2 yr	Active disease	Effective after 3 months
O'Donoghue *et al*, 1978	51	Azathioprine	1 yr	Maintenance, withdrawal	After steroid withdrawal, azathioprine reduces relapses over 1 year
Ursing *et al*, CCDSS, 1982	78	Metronidazole, sulfasalazine	5 mo	Active colitis	Metronidazole slightly more effective; switch S to M good; M to S not
Brynskov *et al*, 1989	71	Cyclosporine	3 mo	Treatment	Cyclosporine 5–7.5 mg/kg; improvement over placebo evident in 2 weeks, and sustained over 3 months
Archembeault *et al*, 1992	305	Cyclosporine	20 mo	Maintenance	Cyclosporine, 4.8 mg/kg/day no better, in some cases worse, than placebo
Prantera *et al*, 1992	125	Mesalamine (Asacol)	1 yr	Maintenance	Those on mesalamine 2.4 grams/day had fewer relapses than with placebo

Implications of the Placebo Response

> Words are, of course, the most powerful drug used by mankind.
> Rudyard Kipling (February 14, 1923)

> One should treat as many patients as possible with a new drug while it still has the power to heal.
> Sir William Osler (1849–1919)

Some further comment on placebos is pertinent. It was noted that the placebo response in the treatment of acute Crohn's disease may be as high as 40 percent. This phenomenon is found in clinical trials of other gastrointestinal disorders, such as the irritable bowel and peptic ulcer. There are important lessons to be drawn from this. First, no costly or potentially harmful diet or pharmacotherapy is acceptable for IBD patients without proof of efficacy through placebo-controlled, double-blind clinical trials.

Second, placebos may be useful in certain circumstances. It is said that if a placebo is to work, the patient should believe that there is a favorable pharmacologic effect. This may not be entirely true, because clinical trials require informed consent to the possible use of placebo, yet those receiving placebo may still improve. In one trial, a small number of neurotic patients improved even when they knew the pills they were given were inert. It seems, therefore, that the symbolic giving of pills has therapeutic effect. The use, therefore, of "logical" placebos, which have a plausible pharmacological rationale, yet do no harm, may be useful in certain circumstances. An example of such a logical placebo might be bran for irregular bowel habit.

The third and probably most important implication of the placebo response is that it reminds us of the beneficial effect of the successful physician–patient encounter. Brody says,

> A clinical approach that makes the illness experience more understandable to the patient, that instills a sense of care and social support, and that will increase the feeling of mastery and control over the course of the illness, will be most likely to create a positive placebo response and to improve symptoms.

Such a positive doctor–patient interaction is indispensable to the management of IBD. Whether or not drugs are employed, careful consideration of the patient's complaints, explanation, and reassurance must be an integral part of any management plan.

SUMMARY

Apart from colectomy in ulcerative colitis, there is no cure for IBD. Much of current therapy is underpinned by controlled trials tempered by a vast wealth of clinical experience. In such vacillating diseases as ulcerative colitis and Crohn's disease, no new treatment can be taken for granted, or general benefit extrapolated from personal experience. Although 5-ASA can be delivered to and is effective in colon disease, we cannot assume that newer preparations released in the small bowel are of actual benefit there. The use of newer yet toxic immunosuppressives in IBD seems logical, but they should not be introduced into clinical practice until properly validated by placebo-controlled, double-blind clinical trials. The failure of such a trial to demonstrate that cyclosporine prevents relapses of Crohn's disease (in fact, it may worsen the disease) is a case in point. In every case both patient and physician must be mindful of the lessons of the placebo response.

Landmark clinical trials of therapy in ulcerative colitis and Crohn's disease are summarized in Tables 24-2 and 24-3. These enterprises result from partnerships between patients and physicians, and their results are indispensable to progress in IBD therapy. Participation by both partners is therefore an important public service.

CHAPTER TWENTY-FIVE

Nutrition and IBD

To eat is human, to digest divine
C. T. Copeland (1860–1952)

Humans must eat to live. Illness may increase the demand for nourishment while depressing appetite. A person with an intestinal illness is further compromised, because eating may exacerbate pain or diarrhea. In small-bowel disease, ingestion, digestion, and absorption of nutrients are impaired; thus in inflammatory bowel disease (IBD), nutrition is a major issue. There are three approaches to nutrition in ulcerative colitis and Crohn's disease: general measures, exceptional measures, and nutrition as treatment. In these chronic illnesses, general measures imply a balanced diet with sufficient calories, including protein, to maintain weight, and adequate vitamins and minerals to sustain healing and correct or prevent deficiencies. Exceptional measures are those necessary to maintain nutrition in an acutely ill patient while he or she undergoes medical or surgical treatment. Such measures include liquid diets, elemental diets, and intravenous feeding. Finally, dietary measures have been employed as treatment. This chapter considers the populations of IBD sufferers at risk, the components of nutrition, and the general, exceptional, and therapeutic applications of nutrition in IBD.

POPULATION AT RISK

Effect of the Illness

The more seriously ill the patient, the greater the nutritional problem. In addition to loss of appetite, one may fear eating, lest it worsen diarrhea or abdominal pain. The disease itself has a catabolic effect; that is, the inflammation, fever, and loss of nutrients from the weeping, inflamed mucosa consume energy and promote weight loss. Depression frequently accompanies chronic illness and further depresses appetite. If the small bowel is diseased, digestion and absorption are impaired. Most nutrients are assimilated in the jejunum, but vitamin B_{12} and bile salts are absorbed exclusively in the ileum. Many years after an ileal resection, vitamin B_{12}–deficiency anemia may occur. Unabsorbed in the ileum, bile salts spill into the colon where they cause diarrhea. Bile salt loss impairs digestion (see the following).

A narrowed segment, usually of the small gut, may become inflamed and block the passage of food. This obstruction causes abdominal pain, distention, and vomiting. In this situation, intravenous fluid replacement is necessary. A fistula, such as an enterocutaneous fistula, may leak intestinal contents and may also require a period of bowel rest and intravenous feeding. An enteroenteral or enterocolic fistula may bypass a long segment of gut so that absorption fails to occur (Figure 14-3). Bacterial overgrowth in a diseased small bowel may also interfere with the digestion and absorption of nutrients.

Effect of Surgery

Repair of tissues after surgery imposes nutritional demands beyond the calorie and protein requirements of the disease itself.

Often the surgery is done in severely ill patients, and is sometimes complicated by sepsis. Furthermore, the surgical patient is unable to eat before, during, and after the procedure; therefore, intravenous feeding becomes the only port of nourishment, until eating can resume. In addition to protein and calories, many vitamins and minerals, such as zinc, are important to the healing process.

Colon surgery, even colectomy, has little residual effect on nutrition; however, if significant segments of small bowel are removed, the patient may be unable to nourish himself orally, and exceptional measures such as defined diets and total parenteral nutrition (TPN) come into play. This is called the short-bowel syndrome, and in extreme cases, home TPN may be the only route to independence.

Effect of Adolescence

Adolescence is a nutritionally demanding period in life. A chronic illness, such as IBD, diverts calories to feed inflammation, sepsis, and repair, and the factors previously described prevent adequate restitution. The bone growth plates (epiphyses) fuse sequentially during adolescence, marking the end of growth in their respective bones. Long-bone growth is completed by late adolescence. Occasionally, growth retardation may be the only presenting manifestation of Crohn's disease, sometimes obscuring the diagnosis. In one study, growth failure occurred in about one third of adolescents with Crohn's. Nutrition during adolescence is critical, and aggressive treatment of the disease is important. In the unusual case of a growth-impaired child with ulcerative colitis who is resistant to drug therapy, colectomy should not be long delayed. The psychological effects of an ileostomy are far outweighed by those of stunted stature. Colectomy ends the disease and permits growth.

A decision to operate is more difficult in Crohn's disease, because cure cannot be guaranteed. Nonetheless, removal of a severely inflamed segment of bowel at a critical point may commence a remission of sufficient duration to permit more growth. Colon may be sacrificed more readily than small bowel. Throughout, aggressive nutritional support must be maintained, even through TPN, if necessary. Nutrients other than calories are also critical for rapid growth. Vitamin D and calcium supplements are needed to prevent rickets, a bone disease of children.

Effect of Pregnancy

The interrelationships of IBD with pregnancy are discussed in Chapter 19. Suffice it to say here that a growing fetus places yet another nutritional demand on a woman with IBD. Here again, adequate supply of minerals and vitamins is as critical as that of calories.

COMPONENTS OF NUTRITION

Calories

The unit of energy is a calorie. In human nutrition, calories are provided by carbohydrate, protein, and fat, which provide 4, 4, and 9 calories per gram, respectively. Calories are essential to such widely divergent functions as growth, muscle contraction, generation of body heat, and tissue repair. They therefore compose the central, but not the only, components of any dietary strategy.

The basic *carbohydrate* units are monosaccharides. Important examples are glucose, fructose, and galactose. Glucose is a source of quick energy and is commonly included in intravenous preparations. These basic sugars are easily absorbed into the blood via the intestinal mucosa. Disaccharides comprise two monosaccharides. Examples are lactose (glucose–galactose), and sucrose (glucose–fructose). On arrival in the small intestine, disaccharides are split into their constituent monosaccharides for quick absorption by their respective disaccharidases (e.g., lactase, sucrase), which are perched on the brush border of the small intestinal epithelium. Adult non-Europeans have low levels of intestinal lactase, and are relatively unable to digest the lactose found in cow's milk and its products. Undigested lactose then travels to the colon, where the local bacteria digest the sugar and release hydrogen (Figure 25-1). The result is a gassy, crampy diarrhea. A diseased or resected small bowel may also maldigest lactose.

There are two groups of more complex dietary carbohydrates, nondigestible and digestible. These are branching chains of glucose. An example of the former is cellulose, an important constituent of dietary fiber. Arriving intact in the colon, it is largely digested by bacteria to produce hydrogen, carbon dioxide, and short-chain fatty acids. These are acetate, butyrate, and propionate, and are important to the nourishment of colonic epithelium (see Chapter 15).

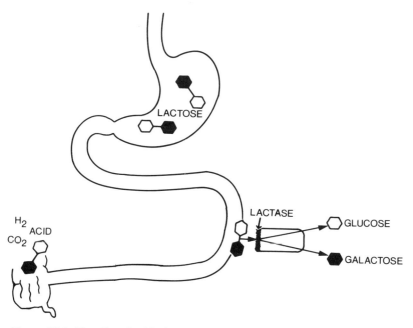

Figure 25-1. The disaccharide lactose consists of two monosaccharides, glucose (white) and galactose (black). This milk sugar is split into its constituent monosaccharides by the small-intestinal mucosal enzyme, lactase, and these are in turn transported to the bloodstream. If the enzyme is deficient, the unabsorbed lactose travels on to the colon, where it is digested by colonic bacteria that release hydrogen, carbon dioxide, and osmotically active metabolites. The result is gas, cramps, and diarrhea.

Digestible carbohydrates include the starches. The pancreatic enzyme amylase, arriving in the duodenum coincident with dietary starch, breaks up the starch, releasing glucose for absorption. Some starches, notably wheat starch, are incompletely digested and provide some fodder for colon bacteria. In contrast, rice starch is more efficiently digested and absorbed. Moreover, in the hurried, contaminated, and inflamed environment of the small intestine in Crohn's disease, all starch may be poorly assimilated.

Whereas carbohydrates provide energy, *proteins* are the structural stuff of which we are made. Protein in bone supports calcium deposition. Muscle protein ensures mobility and strength. Immunoglobulins are blood proteins essential to immunity. In all tissues, proteins form chromosomes, enzymes, and the very skeletons of cells. The basic units are amino acids. Chains of amino acids in various sequences determine the nature of proteins. Albumin is a vital blood protein. It is the principal determinant of the osmotic force of blood. Blood osmolarity attracts water into the bloodstream, and therefore a low blood albumin causes fluid to seep into the tissues. The result is swelling of the ankles, which we call edema. Edema and low albumin levels are therefore good indicators of protein malnutrition.

Proteins are found in meats, vegetables, and grains. They are attacked in a preliminary but not essential way by stomach acid and the enzyme pepsin. The important digestion occurs in the small intestine, where proteolytic enzymes such as trypsin, secreted by the pancreas, break up proteins into their constituent amino acids or short chains called peptides. The latter are further degraded by brush border peptidases in a manner similar to that of the disaccharidases. In small-bowel disease, the amino acid harvest is compromised, despite the increased demands of inflammation and healing. Moreover, protein is lost from the weeping, inflamed mucosa (protein-losing enteropathy). When the body is starved for energy, amino acid stores are sacrificed in the liver to produce glucose. This *gluconeogenesis* can be slowed by the feeding or intravenous infusion of glucose.

Severe protein deficiency obviously manifests as weakness, fatigue, and weight and muscle loss. Hypoalbuminemia and edema have been mentioned. More subtly, the immune system is compromised, impairing resistance to infection. A protein-compromised pancreas may underproduce pancreatic enzymes, further compounding malnutrition. As if the negative effects of IBD were not enough, steroids are catabolic. They favor gluconeogenesis and the breakdown of protein (see Chapter 21). Osteoporosis results from insufficient bone protein, increasing the risk of fractures in later life. In the atmosphere of protein deficiency and lengthy steroid use found in IBD, impaired surgical healing should not be a surprise.

Fats are an important source of energy, and are complex. Because they are calorie intense, they spare carbohydrate, thus permitting a more concentrated diet or intravenous solution. Fat minimizes the blood glucose fluctuations that may accompany high-carbohydrate sources of energy. Fatty acids consist of chains of carbon atoms with an acid radical at one end. The longer the carbon chain, the more water insoluble it becomes. Thus the short-chain fatty acid, butyrate, produced by colon bacteria to feed the colon mucosa, is water soluble. Medium-chain fatty acids are relatively water soluble and easily absorbed by intestinal mucosa. Long-chain fatty acids, such as linoleate, are weakly soluble and require bile salts for solubilization and absorption in the small intestine.

Normally, three fatty acids are attached to a glycerine molecule to form a triglyceride, the principal source of dietary fat. Before assimilation, triglycerides and the closely related phospholipids must be split into their constituents by pancreatic enzymes such as lipase. The freed, weakly water-soluble fatty acids are arranged into micelles, and thereby maintained in solution, through the detergent action of *bile salts*. These fascinating products of liver cholesterol metabolism have water-soluble and fat-soluble properties at opposite poles. In a micelle, the fat-soluble ends of the bile salt molecules are arranged inward and the fatty acids and phospholipids are secured among the bile salts, with their weakly water-soluble acid ends facing outward. Cholesterol and the fat-soluble vitamins huddle in the middle of micelles, which in turn are suspended in intestinal fluid. The micelles thus convey the products of fat digestion to the mucosal brush border for absorption and transport via the lymphatic system to the blood. Medium-chain triglycerides are more water soluble and, once digested, bypass this mechanism; therefore, they are useful in the nourishment of patients with a short bowel or with bile salt insufficiency. The fat-soluble vitamins A, D, E, and K are bile-salt dependent and must be replaced by injection if there is malabsorption of fat.

Bile salts are products of cholesterol metabolism in the liver. The addition of hydroxyl ($-OH$) ions to the cholesterol shell provides the water-soluble aspect of the molecule, which is so essential to the formation of micelles. In bile, bile salts solubilize cholesterol and phospholipids so that they may safely transit the bile ducts and gallbladder to the duodenum. Here the bile salts exert their role in absorption of fat, as previously explained. The bile salts themselves are largely reabsorbed in the ileum and returned to the liver. Disease or resection of the ileum may thus have several important consequences. First, the unabsorbed bile salts escape to the colon where they cause diarrhea. Second, the ensuing depletion of bile salts in the gallbladder favors the dissolution of cholesterol, and gallstones develop. Insufficient bile salts in the small intestine permit malabsorption of fat and fat-soluble vitamins. The loss of fat in the stool (steatorrhea) further exacerbates the diarrhea (see Chapter 14).

Minerals

Iron is a vital constituent of hemoglobin and is essential for red blood cell production by the bone marrow. It is absorbed in the relatively acid medium of the duodenum and stored in the liver, spleen, and bone marrow. The normal body iron store is 3 to 4 grams. Deficiency of iron eventually causes anemia. Although an iron-poor diet (tea and toast) or iron malabsorption due to stomach or intestinal disease occasionally cause iron deficiency, blood loss is a much more likely explanation. In IBD, all three factors may be at work, so adequate iron intake is important, especially in menstruating women. Normally, sufficient iron is provided by regular meat ingestion. Before anemia appears, iron stores may be depleted. This may be assessed by measuring blood levels of iron and the iron-carrying protein ferritin. If blood levels are low, iron replacement is provided through one of the many commercial iron preparations. One normally begins with iron sulfate ($FeSO_4$), 300 milligrams with meals, increasing from one to three a day. Some cannot tolerate $FeSO_4$, so more expensive and less concentrated iron preparations may be tried [e.g., ferrous gluconate, ferrous fumarate, or ferrous sulfate (Slow-Fe)]. Be forewarned that iron-containing drugs color the stool black.

Calcium provides the hardness of bone. Absorbed in the small intestine with the assistance of vitamin D, calcium may be deficient in vitamin D deficiency (rickets, osteomalacia) or dietary calcium deficiency (osteoporosis). Estrogen-deficient postmenopausal women or persons treated with steroids are especially susceptible. Demand for calcium is greatest during adolescence and pregnancy. A major disadvantage of a lactose-free diet is the loss of milk as a source of calcium. If necessary, a commercially available lactase (Lactaid) may be given with milk. Alternatively, yogurt can provide calcium without lactose. Those at risk for calcium deficiency should take calcium supplements such as Os-cal or Tums.

Several other minerals are essential to life. In small-bowel Crohn's, *magnesium* deficiency is common. The trace metal *zinc* is required for wound healing. *Copper, selenium,* and *manganese* are trace elements we seldom consider, but they become critically essential in an exceptional nutrition program in which normal foods are not taken. *Sodium* and *potassium* are important components of blood and indeed all body fluids. Enteral and parenteral feeding must include all of these important minerals.

Vitamins

No aspect of health is more misunderstood than the role of vitamins in human nutrition. Vitamins are coenzymes or catalysts that permit a biochemical reaction. Once a critical intake of a vitamin has been achieved, no excess is of value. Somehow the idea is abroad that if a little vitamin is good, then a lot is better. In some cases, this notion is harmless. Vitamin B_{12}, for example, may be given in great excess without harm and without much expense; however, an overdose of vitamins A or D can be fatal. Perhaps the very term *vitamin* is at fault. These substances are essential metabolic facilitators, not pick-me-ups. In healthy people, they are adequately acquired from a normal diet.

Vitamin A is a fat-soluble vitamin that may be deficient in certain malabsorption states. The result may be night-blindness and dry, scaly skin. *Vitamin D* is essential for absorption of calcium and its deposition in bone. Deficiency produces rickets in children and osteomalacia in adults. An overdose may cause a fatal rise in serum calcium. *Vitamin K* is another fat-soluble vitamin needed for the production of some blood-clotting factors in the liver. Deficiency may cause bruising and bleeding, and is detected by a blood-clotting test called the prothrombin time. The last fat-soluble vitamin, *vitamin E*, is seldom important in IBD.

There are several vitamins B. *Thiamine* (B_1) deficiency is responsible for beriberi, a disease of heart, brain, and other tissues, which is commonly seen in the Third World. Lack of *riboflavin* (B_2) causes skin lesions, notably around the angle of the mouth (cheilosis). Pellagra is due to *niacin* (B_3) deficiency. Its many manifestations include sore tongue, diarrhea, mental illness, and a sun-sensitive dermatitis. Sore tongue, anemia, and nerve and muscle damage are found with *pyridoxine* (B_6) deficiency. *Folic acid* (B_9) and *vitamin B_{12}* deficiencies most notably cause a sore tongue and anemia, but have other effects as well. Low blood folate may be seen with insufficient dietary folic acid, malabsorption, or the antifolate effects of sulfasalazine. Inadequate *vitamin C* is responsible for scurvy, which is characterized by bleeding into tissues. There may be bruising or typically bleeding into hair follicles (see James Lind's description of scurvy in Chapter 24). All of these deficiencies are easily prevented. Clearly any nutritional program must include vitamins.

GENERAL MEASURES

Eat what you want and let the food fight it out inside.
Mark Twain (1835–1910)

This sentiment could be the motto of the coke and chips generation, but it is true that the human gut is remarkably efficient at extracting what the body needs from a normal, no-frills diet. To be sure, and not just for IBD, one needs to avoid junk food, inadequate dietary fiber, saturated fats, and excess alcohol. Normally for inactive or mild disease, no other dietary considerations are necessary in IBD. A dietician may be employed to assist a young patient achieve a well-balanced diet. In accordance with a normal appetite, three meals a day, at least one with meat; dairy products; and fruits and vegetables should provide the necessary nutrients.

Special circumstances may dictate special provisions. Chronic blood loss may necessitate iron replacement. Exacerbations of IBD may depress appetite, yet increase caloric need. If possible, food intake should be sufficient to prevent weight loss. If lactose intolerant, one must avoid milk. Then calcium must be supplied by yogurt or calcium supplements, especially in the young, the pregnant, and the menopausal. The proscription of the wheat protein *gluten* is essential in celiac disease, which rarely may coexist with IBD. Body folic acid stores are sufficient for 1 month, so supplements should be provided if prolonged fasting is imposed by disease, especially if the folic acid antagonists sulfasalazine or 6-mercaptopurine (6-MP) are being used. A long-standing ileal resection may necessitate vitamin B_{12} injections. The B_{12} requirement is predictable by means of a Schilling test, which measures B_{12} absorption capacity (Chapter 27). Malabsorption or bile salt deficiencies necessitate vitamins A, D, and K replacement. If in doubt, a multivitamin preparation with about 400 international units of vitamin D may be taken daily, especially in the winter, when fresh fruit, vegetables, and sunshine are limited. Such supplements are advisable in adolescence and pregnancy. More than one vitamin pill or capsule is unnecessary, and many may be harmful.

Contemporary IBD patients are bombarded by conflicting and unsubstantiated dietary advice. Books promise cure if only one will follow a natural diet. The word "natural" often owes much to the literary license of the author. Fringe practitioners, like their forerunners the snake oil salesmen, advocate all sorts of special diets for IBD. Some are so restrictive as to cause malnutrition. One young man with known ulcerative colitis was admitted to hospital with a 20-pound weight loss and worsening disease, having been per-

suaded by a diet book that restricting his intake to special carbohydrates would cure his colitis. The IBD sufferer is well advised to
beware these traps and if in doubt, discuss the matter with a
physician, who may direct him or her to a qualified nutritionist.

EXCEPTIONAL MEASURES

Active IBD may impair the employment of the general measures
discussed previously. Decreased food intake may result from poor
appetite, small-bowel malabsorption, obstructing lesions, and fistulas. Increased nutritional demand is a consequence of inflammation, sepsis, and fever. Such circumstances have stimulated the
development of defined formula diets and intravenous feeding
techniques. All these feedings contain the essential calories, minerals, and vitamins.

Defined Formula Diets

These are liquid diets that provide all the essential nutrients.
Unlike intravenous feeding, oral feeds may be given to outpatients.
They nourish the gut mucosa, which is likely to atrophy with
disuse. Diarrhea may occur when refeeding a rested gut. Theoretically, these liquid diets are assimilated in the small gut, resting
the colon, and should be more easily passed through strictured,
inflamed bowel. A large number of either polymeric or elemental
commercial preparations are available. The contents of polymeric
diets require some degree of digestion before they can be absorbed.
Some (e.g., Sustacal, Mead Johnson) have lactose and dietary
residue, whereas others, such as Isocal (Mead Johnson) are lactose
and residue free and have an osmolarity similar to that of blood. The
debate about the relative merits of the many polymeric diets is
beyond our scope here. The features that distinguish them from the
elemental diets are their relative palatability, their relative cheap-
ness, and their intact protein, which requires digestion. If necessary,
these diets may be delivered by a fine nasogastric tube. In recogni-

tion of the importance of dietary fiber to nutrition generally, fiber is added to some polymeric diets in the form of soy carbohydrates.

Elemental Diets

Elemental diets (Vital, Vivonex, Tolerex) contain elements that require little or no digestion. Their development owes much to the space industry, since stool and colon gas production create awkward moments in an astronaut's suit. Protein is supplied as amino acids or short amino acid chains called peptides, which are often hydrolysates of whole proteins. Fat is provided as medium-chain triglycerides. These constituents are in many respects ideal in IBD for certain situations. They should be rapidly absorbed in a shortened or diseased gut, without need of digestion. Gas-forming colon bacteria are deprived of fuel. The minimal residue of an elemental diet should maximize bowel rest yet maintain mucosal nutrition; however, the disadvantages are expense and unpalatability. A new product called Peptamen seems to have a more acceptable taste. Sometimes these liquid diets must be administered through a nasogastric tube.

Parenteral (Intravenous) Nutrition

Bowel rest is a time-honored treatment of acute IBD. The efficacy of such treatment is not established, but often the patient's symptoms permit no other course. A simple intravenous solution contains sodium, chloride, and/or glucose. The latter may provide a few hundred calories a day, thereby slowing protein breakdown (gluconeogenesis). Vitamins, potassium, and other elements may be added as necessary, and the intravenous line is a handy port for drugs such as prednisolone and antibiotics. In a previously well person, such an approach may do for a few days while therapy is begun, symptoms are relieved, and until oral feeding can be reestablished. Longer fasting periods require more aggressive intravenous feeding.

A simple intravenous line may be installed in an arm vein (Figure 25-2). Such peripheral venous infusion is possible if the infusate is isotonic, that is, it has the same osmotic force as blood. This may be achieved through the use of fat as the principal nonprotein source of energy. A commercial fat emulsion called Intralipid is available for this purpose. This is not an ideal imitation of the normal diet, and it depends on healthy peripheral veins, which are sometimes rare in chronic illness. It does, however, avoid the risks of thrombosis or sepsis that accompany the use of a central line.

A central venous line permits infusion of hypertonic solutions and therefore more flexibility (Figure 25-3). One can more closely mimic the balance of carbohydrate, protein, and fat found in a normal diet. In addition to the vitamins and minerals provided with the feeding solutions, periodic addition of vitamins K and B_{12} are important. Aseptic care of the central line is crucial if this port of entry is to be preserved, and sepsis or major vein thrombosis, avoided.

Rarely, sequential operations may leave the patient with a short bowel, incapable of adequate nutrient assimilation. If an elemental

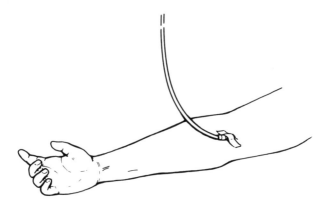

Figure 25-2. Peripheral intravenous line. This may be a port for intravenous feeding.

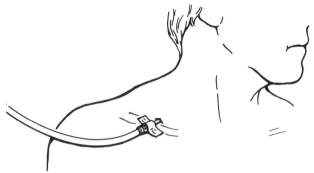

Figure 25-3. Central venous line. A large-bore catheter into the great veins of the neck serves as a port for total parenteral nutrition (TPN).

diet is unsuccessful, even by continuous nasogastric tube infusion, home TPN may be the only means by which independent living can be restored. A permanent central silicone catheter is carefully placed in the superior vena cava via a major neck vein, such as the subclavian. A special attachment permits the short-bowel patient to attach presupplied nutrient packages to the catheter and infuse at night, thus freeing him or her for the next day's activities. A small oral intake may be taken as tolerated. In Crohn's disease, less aggressive surgical practices should make a short-bowel syndrome requiring home TPN less common (see Chapter 26).

DIET AS TREATMENT

Good nutrition permits healing while other measures, such as drugs and surgery, attack the disease. Beyond this, some believe that certain dietary measures are themselves therapeutic. The bases for this belief are the notions of bowel rest and that a luminal factor initiates the inflammation (Chapter 6). Therapeutic diets have received more attention for Crohn's disease than for ulcerative colitis.

The efficacy of bowel rest remains to be proven. It certainly relieves symptoms during an attack, especially those due to obstruction. This notion makes sense intuitively. After all, a broken arm is immobilized to permit healing; so it should be with the gut. More problematic is the concept of a luminal factor. Unlike the case of gluten in celiac disease, no such factor has been discovered for IBD. Furthermore, such a factor could be bacterial, rather than dietary.

Total parenteral nutrition offers the most complete bowel rest, and should eliminate any putative dietary luminal factor. Some reports claim improved healing of fistulas and abscesses with TPN, but clinical trials have failed to demonstrate effectiveness in Crohn's disease itself, independent of TPN's nutritional value. It is clear that if TPN is employed as treatment, no oral feeding should be permitted, lest the bowel-rest and luminal hypotheses be compromised.

In Europe, there is interest in an elemental diet as a treatment for Crohn's disease. Like TPN, such a diet provides some bowel rest and eliminates whole protein as a possible luminal factor. Such an approach is easier, safer, and cheaper, and should maximize nutrition of the intestinal mucosa. If an elemental diet (e.g., Vivonex, Tolerex, Vital) is unpalatable, it may be delivered via a feeding tube. Some patients learn to insert such a tube themselves. Nevertheless, there is little to make one believe that an elemental diet should succeed where TPN has not, unless it is through some local mucosal nutrition.

A small (12 patients, 2 dropouts) therapeutic trial by O'Morain in 1984 found an elemental diet to be as effective in the treatment of an exacerbation of Crohn's disease as prednisolone. Now practicing in Dublin, he successfully employs this technique on patients both in and out of the hospital. A larger German trial using short-chain peptides rather than amino acids showed an elemental diet to be less effective than standard therapy with steroids and sulfasalazine. Although this approach deserves further study, it has not become a common practice in North America. It may be used, however, *with* steroid therapy.

Another therapeutic approach is based on the notion that some patients are hypersensitive (not allergic) to some foods. Cambridge doctors report the usefulness to some Crohn's patients of an elimination diet that systematically tests wheat, eggs, and milk products. Unfortunately this work has not been replicated elsewhere. If effective at all, it must benefit only a few. In ulcerative colitis, a fish-oil diet has been proposed, because of its effect on the mucosal production of prostaglandins and leukotrienes. Such treatments, although based on legitimate hypotheses, should be regarded as experimental.

"We are what we eat," say some. True to a point, this cliché provides license for quack diets for which proponents have the temerity to claim cure. Make no mistake, in IBD this is a cruel hoax. The reality is that no diet is proven curative, and those profiting from the employment of fanciful diets eschew any suggestion of scientific testing. Some can be dangerous and should not be adopted in IBD without expert advice.

SUMMARY

Good nutrition is important for everyone. The nutrients are calories provided by carbohydrate, protein, and fat, and adequate, but not excess minerals and vitamins. The patient with IBD may have special needs. Inflammation, sepsis, fever, and nutrient loss from the inflamed gut increase caloric demand. Chronic blood loss depletes iron. Poor intake of calcium and vitamin D causes rickets in children and osteomalacia or osteoporosis in adults, the latter compounded by chronic steroid therapy. Small-bowel disease is especially likely to imperil nutrition. Loss of ileal function may cause vitamin B_{12} malabsorption, diarrhea, and malassimilation of fat and fat-soluble vitamins through bile salt loss. Extensive jejunal disease promotes malabsorption of fluid and almost all other elements of nutrition. Obstruction, inflammation, and short bowel require exceptional measures, such as a polymeric or elemental oral feeding, which may need to be delivered by nasogastric tube. Another exceptional measure is TPN. Adolescence, pregnancy, infection, and surgery impose extra demands. The employment of diet as treatment is controversial, and TPN appears to little alter the course of the disease once nutrition has been attended to. The enthusiasm for an elemental diet in the British Isles has not caught on elsewhere. The field is wide open for quack diets, so buyer beware!

CHAPTER TWENTY-SIX

Surgery in IBD

Diseases desperate grown
By desperate appliance are relieved,
Or not at all.
Shakespeare, *Hamlet* (Act IV, Sc ii)

When the medical management of inflammatory bowel disease (IBD) fails, or a serious complication intervenes, we are fortunate to have a surgical option. Skillful and timely operative intervention against a background of optimal medical care should provide acceptable functioning for most IBD sufferers. Yet patients frequently labor under the shadow of several myths and misconceptions about surgery, and these may interfere with its expedient employment. These misconceptions take two forms. Many patients fear the consequences of surgery, especially an ileostomy or colostomy, and the effect of such a device on their "personhood." Others, especially those with Crohn's disease, look to surgery as a panacea— a physical and symbolic extirpation of the disease. This chapter explains the surgical procedures commonly employed in IBD, and dispels the misconceptions.

Although ulcerative colitis and Crohn's disease have many similar attributes, especially if only the colon is involved, their surgical management is not the same. The fundamental difference is that, in the case of ulcerative colitis, the disease may be cured by colectomy. Whatever the ultimate disposition of the terminal ileum may be (an ileostomy, an ileorectal anastomosis, or an ileal pouch–anal anastomosis), with no colon, one can have no colitis. This is not the case in Crohn's disease, which can affect any level of the gut from mouth to anus. No reasonable surgical approach can completely remove the disease, and recurrence following operation is very likely. Despite this, the risk of cancer complicating Crohn's disease is much less than that with ulcerative colitis (Chapter 17). These factors dictate a more conservative approach to surgery in Crohn's disease. When a stricture, fistula, or intractable disease indicates surgery, the minimal operation is done in order to preserve as much functioning bowel as possible. Furthermore, the virtual inevitability of recurrence of Crohn's disease mitigates against an ileal pouch–anal anastomosis following colectomy. Thus, surgery in ulcerative colitis may be said to be curative, whereas in Crohn's disease, it is palliative; that is, it alleviates without curing.

SURGERY FOR ULCERATIVE COLITIS

Indications

The indications for surgery in ulcerative colitis can be elective, imperative, or emergency (Table 26-1). When disease continues despite optimal medical management so that growth, employment, or social integrity is threatened, patient and physician eventually arrive at the conclusion that colectomy is a better option. Often this conclusion is hastened by lengthy dependence on drugs, especially steroids, or the increasing risk of cancer after 10 to 15 years of disease. Some of the extraintestinal manifestations of ulcerative colitis, such as colitic arthritis or erythema nodosum, follow the same course as ulcerative colitis. If these are severe, colectomy may be helpful. Others, such as pyoderma gangrenosum, may or may not improve with surgery, and still others, namely rheumatoid spondylitis or sclerosing cholangitis, pursue an independent course, unaffected by surgery. The moment of operation is elective, and it

TABLE 26-1
Ulcerative Colitis: Indications for Surgery

A. Elective: Intractable colitis
   Growth retardation
   Social dysfunction
   Employment dysfunction
   Steroid dependence
   Severe extraintestinal manifestations: colitic arthritis, uveitis, erythema
      nodosum (pyoderma gangrenosum[a])
B. Imperative: Cancer prophylaxis
   Colonic stricture
   Intraluminal mass
   Dysplasia on colonic biopsy
   Long-standing pancolitis
C. Emergency: Complicated ulcerative colitis
   Fulminant colitis
   Toxic megacolon
   Perforation
   Severe hemorrhage

[a]A doubtful indication.

is ultimately the patient's decision to proceed; thus, he or she must be fully informed of the consequences of surgery versus continued medical therapy.

When cancer threatens, colon removal becomes imperative. Such a situation occurs when a stricture or mass is found in the colon, or when colon mucosal biopsies indicate severe dysplasia, a precancerous lesion (see Chapter 17). In extensive colitis, the cancer risk increases after 10 years. In Copenhagen, 31 percent of all ulcerative colitis patients had a colectomy by 18 years. In those considering elective colectomy, concern about cancer may facilitate the decision.

When a serious complication of ulcerative colitis intervenes, there is no choice but to remove the colon as soon as possible. In some cases fulminant disease may be treated medically. This may be desirable in a new case in which the patient has not been prepared psychologically for surgery; however, in most of these, colectomy

is eventually required. With toxic megacolon, massive hemorrhage, or perforation, delay is not an option.

Colectomy

In the early 1900s, ileostomy was performed on patients with
ulcerative colitis. The aim was to rest the colon for a period of
time with a view to restoration of gut continuity when the colitis
remitted. It soon became evident, however, that in many cases, the
ileostomy was permanent. Thus a two-stage operation became the
standard: ileostomy followed later by a total colectomy. It was not
until the 1950s that a one-stage colectomy and ileostomy became
routine practice. Occasionally in a very ill patient, a subtotal
colectomy and ileostomy is performed as an emergency. In this
case, the rectum may be removed at a later date.

Early on, the results of surgery for ulcerative colitis were poor,
mainly because the decision to intervene was delayed. Even now, the
results are best when surgery is done electively, rather than in the
presence of very severe or complicated ulcerative colitis.

The colectomy itself is usually uncomplicated and straightfor-
ward. The terminal ileum is transected, and the intraabdominal
colon dissected from its supporting mesentery, nerves, and blood
vessels. The colon is then removed, leaving 15 centimeters of rectum
in the pelvis. The open end of the ileum is then brought up to the
abdominal wall, and an ileostomy is created (Figure 26-2).

Once the decision to perform a colectomy has been made, the
principal issue facing the surgeon and patient is what to do with
the disconnected terminal ileum. There are four possible choices;
ileorectal anastomosis with retention of the rectum; ileostomy;
continent ileostomy; or ileal pouch–anal anastomosis.

Ileorectal Anastomosis

In an effort to avoid a permanent ileostomy and retain continence, abdominal (subtotal) colectomy and ileorectal anastomosis

(Figure 26-1) has been advocated in selected cases. With this operation, the anal sphincter and pelvic floor muscles are retained to control the flow of stool and air. Because no pelvic dissection is required, there is little risk of postoperative sexual or urinary dysfunction. This surgery requires a capacious rectum capable of storing stool, and quiescent disease to ensure healing at the anastomosis. It is not possible if the rectum is scarred or narrowed by the disease (see Figure 10-3), or in the face of severe active colitis. Even so, anastomotic leaks may cause a significant postoperative illness (morbidity). If ileorectal anastomosis is successful, subsequent bowel motions usually occur four to five times per day.

The principal disadvantage of this operation is that it is not a cure. Continuing rectal disease usually requires local and systemic treatment, often with steroids. One fourth to one half of these cases eventually need removal of the rectum, and until then the specter of rectal malignancy remains. With these hazards, few contemporary surgeons will offer such a procedure for the treatment of ulcerative colitis. In certain cases, an established ileorectal anastomosis may be converted to an ileal pouch. In Crohn's colitis, sometimes the rectum is spared, making ileorectal anastomosis feasible. In this case, there is little risk of cancer in the retained rectum; however, in the event of a rectal recurrence, a permanent ileostomy may be required.

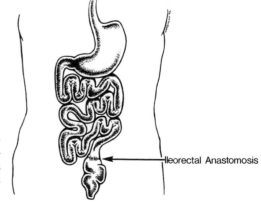

Figure 26-1. Ileorectal anastomosis. After removal of the colon (subtotal colectomy), the terminal ileum is joined to the rectum, which is still susceptible to recurrence of IBD.

Ileorectal Anastomosis

Ileostomy

The currently performed ileostomy (Figure 26-2) was designed by Brooke. In this procedure, the severed end of the ileum is pulled through a small incision in the abdominal wall. It is everted and made to "pout" 1 to 2 centimeters above the skin where it is stitched in place. A close-fitting ileostomy appliance then prevents fecal contamination and excoriation of the skin. The Brooke ileostomy has been the standard since it was reported in the *Lancet* in 1952. The important innovations that made ileostomy acceptable, however, were the development of reliable ileostomy appliances in the 1930s, with improvements in the 1980s. Current stomal appliances have a plastic faceplate, which is held to the skin about the opening (stoma) by a special cement. This apparatus is easily changed and maintained by the patient once he or she has been properly trained. The collecting bag must be emptied four or five times a day, but the faceplate is changed only once a week. Clearly the enterostomal therapist is a key person. This professional teaches ileostomy management, advises on the selection of appliances, and preoperatively even helps select the site of the stoma on the abdominal wall. This choice of site is important and is generally in the right

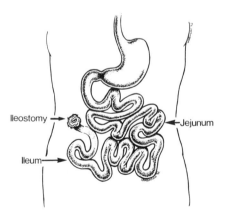

Figure 26-2. Ileostomy. The colon has been removed (total colectomy), and the severed end of the ileum is sewn through the abdominal wall.

lower area of the abdomen so as to fit beneath underwear or bathing suit.

Total proctocolectomy has a small, but significant mortality, which rises sharply if the patient is very ill to begin with. The perineum where the anus is sealed is a notoriously disadvantageous site for healing. It may take weeks to months to close completely. As many as 10 percent of patients later require a second operation for small-bowel obstruction at the ileostomy. Newer surgical techniques minimize the risk of damage to the sacral nerves, so sexual and urinary function are usually retained.

The normal ileostomy effluent is 200 to 700 milliliters per day, and over time becomes less liquid, even formed. The odor is not fecal, and is easily contained by the appliance. Because the usual water- and sodium-retaining capacity of the colon is lost, an intervening diarrheal illness may result in exaggerated dehydration and sodium loss. In such an event, especially in a hot climate, intravenous water and salt restoration may be necessary.

Compared to the handicaps of chronic ulcerative colitis and steroids, the quality of life with an ileostomy is very good (see Chapter 18). Lack of fecal control is cited as a major disadvantage, yet for veterans of ulcerative colitis, the stomal appliance may provide an independence they have long since forgotten. Indeed, it is not rare for some patients with a temporary ileostomy, pending an ileal pouch–anal anastomosis, to be so much relieved that they forego the second surgery. Ultimately, however, one must remove the remaining diseased rectum.

Ileostomy permits a normal life. This includes sexual activity, childbearing, and normal employment. Body-image difficulties are greater in young people, especially if the operation is an emergency and there is little time preoperatively for teaching and adjustment. This is more than just vanity. Many fear the appliance will interfere with marriage, childbearing, or even employment. Laborers may experience herniation of the ileum through the stoma with heavy lifting, but otherwise disability is remarkably slight.

In one survey, 95 percent of respondents expressed satisfaction with their ileostomy, but 40 percent would like a change. Despite the satisfaction, appliances are a drag; thus, surgeons have been motivated to design other dispositions for the ileum. The two most notable are the Koch continent ileostomy, and Park's ileal pouch–anal anastomosis.

Continent Ileostomy (Koch)

The object of this ileostomy technique is to provide continence with patient control of evacuation, without the need of an appliance. The end 45 centimeters of ileum is used to fashion the pouch reservoir. The pouch itself consists of two 15-centimeter segments sewn together as a "J." The last 15 centimeters is used to make a one-way "nipple" valve within the "J," which obstructs the fecal flow. Over time, the pouch capacity increases. The patient evacuates the pouch at his or her convenience by means of a catheter inserted five or six times a day through the one-way valve into the pouch. Only a small pad applied flush with the skin is necessary to cover the opening (stoma).

The operative technique is difficult, and surgical revision of the Koch pouch is necessary in as many as 50 percent of cases. Hemorrhage, valve slippage, obstruction, fistula, and sepsis are common, and pouchitis occurs in about one third of cases (Chapter 15). Despite these many setbacks and sometimes repeated surgery, continence is eventually achieved in most cases. A Brooke ileostomy can be converted to a continent ileostomy if desired. The procedure should not be done in patients with Crohn's disease, in whom recurrence at the stomal site is likely. Nowadays, the desire for continence is more satisfactorily fulfilled by an ileal pouch–anal anastomosis, which has largely replaced the continent ileostomy.

Ileal Pouch–Anal Anastomosis

Clearly, the optimal disposition of the ileum following total colectomy is an ileoanal anastomosis. Simple suture of the severed ileum to the anus is not feasible, however, because there is no reservoir to replace the rectum. The result would be a constant need to defecate (15 to 20 times per day).

A British surgeon, Sir Alan Parks, developed a technique that preserved anal musculature and fashioned an ileal pouch reservoir or neorectum. The ileal pouch–anal anastomosis (Figure 26-3) has also been called an *ileoanal anastomosis*, or more awkwardly, reconstructive proctectomy. To begin this operation, the ileum must be mobilized from its position in the right lower quadrant of the abdomen. Its nerve and blood supply must be carefully preserved. In a manner similar to that of the Koch pouch, a "J" reservoir is fashioned with the ileum. The abdominal colectomy is completed down to the pelvic floor muscles surrounding the lower 5 centimeters of rectum and anus. From below, the diseased mucosa is stripped from these muscles, while preserving anal sphincter function. The newly fashioned ileal reservoir is seated in and above the anal muscles and opened through the anus. A temporary "loop" ileostomy is usually placed in the right lower abdomen to decompress the gut and permit pouch healing over a 3-month period.

Techniques have improved with experience over the last decade, and the results of this operation are very acceptable. In an ill or undecided patient, a two-stage procedure (not including the ileostomy closure) may be planned. Colectomy and ileostomy are done, and the anorectum is preserved for construction of a future ileal pouch. Some patients may stop at this point, relieved at

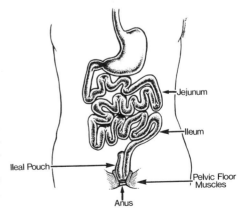

Figure 26-3. Ileal pouch–anal anastomosis. The colon has been removed, and the rectal mucosa stripped from the rectal muscle. A pouch is fashioned from the end of the ileum and seated in the anorectal muscles.

Jejunum

Ileum

Ileal Pouch

Pelvic Floor Muscles

Anus

last to be free of symptoms. Nonetheless, disease may continue in the rectal mucosa. Because Crohn's disease may involve all layers of the gut, and recurrence in the anus is likely, an ileal pouch–anal anastomosis is unsuitable for this condition.

Operative and postoperative complications occur in about one fourth of cases and include small-bowel obstruction, pelvic abscess, wound infection, and urinary infection. When the ileostomy is closed, small-bowel obstruction or leak may occur at the suture line. In about 5 percent, anorectal infection becomes a serious problem, and conversion to a permanent ileostomy is required. An inflammation of the ileoanal pouch called *pouchitis* occurs any time after surgery in as many as one third of patients. It is usually treated successfully with metronidazole (Chapter 15). About 1 percent of patients have some sexual dysfunction, such as retrograde ejaculation or impotence in men and dyspareunia (painful intercourse) in women. These are usually temporary, and less common than those seen after surgical removal of the rectum for cancer. Sexual dysfunction should lessen as technique improves.

Despite these drawbacks, 95 percent of patients express satisfaction with their neorectum. Quality-of-life studies show superior performance in those with an ileal pouch–anal anastomosis, compared to those with the Brooke ileostomy. The former have significant advantages in the performance of daily activities, and are more active in sports and sexual relationships. Normal pregnancy and even delivery at term are possible with the pelvic pouch. In one series, howover, 9 of 20 women had Caesarian deliveries to avoid anal sphincter damage.

What, Then, Should Be Done with the Terminal Ileum?

Ileorectal anastomosis is not a safe procedure for ulcerative colitis because of poor healing where the ileum is joined to the diseased rectum, continuing rectal disease, and the lifelong risk of rectal cancer. On exceptional occasions it may be employed in very young or very old patients if the rectal disease is quiescent. It may be acceptable in certain cases of Crohn's disease. It seems that the Koch pouch offers little advantage over a standard ileostomy and is fraught with many technical difficulties. The ileal pouch–anal anastomosis has rendered it obsolete. The practical choice then lies between a standard ileostomy and an ileal pouch–anal anastomosis.

A surgical neorectum is contraindicated if there is any possibility of Crohn's disease. In indeterminate colitis, the decision may be postponed by the performance of an abdominal colectomy and ileostomy, leaving the rectum in place. The second, or pouch, stage is then aborted if the pathologist determines that the removed colon was affected by Crohn's rather than ulcerative colitis. In this case, an ileorectal anastomosis may be contemplated if the rectum recovers. An older patient whose social and body image are established, and whose reproduction is completed, might decide to waive the extra trouble and accept a permanent ileostomy. In an emergency, the surgeon must perform a lifesaving subtotal colectomy and ileostomy, and avoid lengthening the procedure through cosmetic considerations. The risks are already high if the patient is ill, septic, and malnourished. Here again, ileal pouch or ileorectal anastomosis may be considered on recovery.

The social disadvantages of colectomy, even with an ileostomy, are greatly exaggerated, and no patient colectomized for ulcerative colitis wants his or her colon back. Nonetheless, in a young, otherwise healthy patient with quiescent disease, a one-stage ileal pouch–anal anastomosis performed by a qualified surgeon seems well worth the attempt.

SURGERY FOR CROHN'S DISEASE

For ulcerative colitis, surgery is definitive, curative, and final. The only decisions center around timing, and the final disposition of the terminal ileum. In contrast, Crohn's disease surgery is tentative, palliative, and usually not final. Because the disease involves the whole gut, recurrence is the rule; cure is exceptional. Although surgery is necessary to deal with the complications of Crohn's, it little alters the natural history of the disease. In one study, recurrence of Crohn's disease proximal to the anastomosis was endo-scopically observed within 3 months in two thirds of patients after ileocolic resection. In one third, symptoms also returned within that period. In many respects, the recurrent disease resembles the original. Nonetheless, 80 percent of Crohn's patients require sur-gery, and the symptoms may be alleviated for a long period. Earlier operators widely excised the diseased bowel in an attempt to eradicate the disease. Contemporary surgeons have learned to delay surgery as long as possible, and then do the minimal procedure needed to deal with complications, while preserving as much functioning gut as possible (see also Chapters 13 and 14).

Resection

If Crohn's disease is confined to a short segment of badly damaged gut, and operation is indicated, then removal of a segment of bowel (resection) may be considered. The indications may be an obstructing stricture or narrow segment, massive hemorrhage, or fistula with or without an abscess. The colon is relatively expend-able, so a total or segmental colectomy may be done for severe Crohn's colitis. Ileorectal anastomosis is possible if the rectum is spared. If not, then the colectomy must be total with an accompany-ing ileostomy. Ileal pouches are contraindicated in Crohn's disease. Occasionally the left colon and rectum are removed, and the patient is left with a colostomy. Such retention of the right colon is of little value to the patient, and a colostomy is more difficult to manage than an ileostomy because of the effluent's solid consistency and fecal odor. Recurrence of Crohn's in the remaining colon is very common, and may eventually force an ileostomy.

Because of its absorptive function, small-bowel preservation is a predominant consideration. Earlier and repeated surgical attempts to eradicate the disease often resulted in the short-bowel syndrome and serious malnutrition. In severe, intractable ileocecal disease with or without a stricture or fistula, respite may be achieved with ileocecal resection and anastomosis to the ascending or transverse colon (Figure 26-4). If less than 60 to 100 centimeters of ileum is

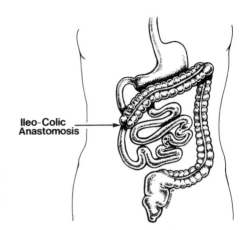

Ileo-Colic Anastomosis →

Figure 26-4. Ileocolic resection. The terminal ileum and cecum have been removed, and the remaining ileum is joined to the transverse colon (ileotransverse or ileocolic anastomosis).

removed, the fat- and vitamin B_{12}-absorbing function is preserved, although bile salt loss into the colon and diarrhea may sometimes ensue. Similarly, a small segment of jejunum may be resected without compromise of absorptive function. If at all possible, repeated or large resections must be avoided.

Minimal Surgery

A common complication of Crohn's disease is a stricture of the small bowel, or much less commonly, the colon. Superimposed edema and inflammation may further narrow the gut and precipitate an episode of bowel obstruction. This may subside as the inflammation is controlled by steroids, and the gut is decompressed through nasogastric suction. If not, surgery must be done. Resection of a single stricture is practical. However, if there are many strictures, rather than resect all the diseased area, the surgeon will try to preserve as much functioning small bowel as possible. This may be accomplished through stricturoplasty, whereby a stricture is surgically widened with no loss of intestine. Minimal surgery also applies to infection. With the guidance of computerized tomography (CT) or ultrasound, some abscesses may be drained by a radiologist employing a long needle.

Perianal Crohn's Disease Surgery

Perianal Crohn's disease presents some of the most frustrating problems in surgery. Local abscesses, fistulas, strictures, and ulcers may be chronic, recurring, and defiant of several surgical approaches. The surgeon confines treatment therefore, to drainage of pus, and strives to maintain sphincter function and patency. Some fistulas may be opened. The antibiotic metronidazole may reduce pain and discharge of pus and can be used for prolonged periods (Chapter 23). Sometimes a colostomy or ileostomy is necessary to divert the fecal flow and permit healing. Too often, this is unsuccessful, and the ostomy becomes permanent.

SUMMARY

In ulcerative colitis, colectomy is curative. The principal issues are timing and the disposition of the terminal ileum. The informed patient may play the major, indeed the pivotal, role in these decisions, short of emergencies. He or she can be equipped to weigh the risks and benefits. Unfortunately, the situation is very different in Crohn's disease, in which surgery is seldom curative. Surgeons have learned to delay, to preserve as much gut as possible, and to refrain from operating on all but the most intractable or complicated disease. Thus, the time, and the type of surgery are usually dictated by circumstances. To be sure, the patient must consent to operation, but the tactical decisions in Crohn's surgery are usually borne by the surgeon, who must be prepared to deal with unprecedented situations.

CHAPTER TWENTY-SEVEN

Investigating the Angry Gut

A patient with an inflamed gut must undergo some tests, first for diagnosis, and subsequently to monitor progress of the disease. The indications for these tests, which vary greatly from case to case, have been discussed in previous chapters. Tests are expensive, and sometimes uncomfortable. They are necessary to determine the presence and extent of gut involvement; however, once diagnosis is established, tests should be performed only when the results will influence treatment. An understanding of the principles and methods of these tests may make them less awesome.

ENDOSCOPY

Modern endoscopy has been made possible by fiberoptic technology. When viewing a water fountain, you may have noticed that light from the base of the fountain follows a stream of water through its arc. A single glass fiber has the same property, so light that enters the fiber at one end follows the fiber through bends and loops to exit at the other. By arranging many fine glass fibers such that their relationship to one another is identical at both ends, one may transmit an image through the bundle. A gastroscope, which transmits light through its length into the duodenum by one fiber bundle, may thus transmit the image of the lining of the duodenum back through another bundle around the many twists and turns of the stomach and esophagus to the examiner's eye.

The technology of endoscopy is still evolving. Through microchips it is now possible for physicians, assistants, and even patients to view the endoscopic image on a television monitor. Videotapes are possible. This technology reduces dependency on delicate fiberoptic bundles, and industry policy is already planning obsolescence for the standard fiberoptic instruments. *Sic transit gloria!* This high-tech equipment is costly, and does not necessarily represent a significant advance over fiberoptics in the care of patients with inflammatory bowel disease (IBD).

Modern endoscopes are equipped with cables controlled by dials (on the handle of the instrument), which move the tip of the scope to the required attitude. There is at least one tube within the instrument through which intestinal juices may be suctioned, or biopsy forceps, cautery, and other devices may be deployed. Not only are these instruments useful in diagnosis, but a number of operations also may be done via the endoscope such as biopsy, cautery of a bleeding lesion, polyp removal, or foreign-body retrieval.

Esophagogastroduodenoscopy

A fiberoptic gastroscope is shown in Figure 27-1. The device to which it is attached contains the external light source and provides suction and air pressure. The shaft is little more than a meter in length and has a diameter similar to that of a pencil. It is quite flexible and light.

A patient undergoing esophagogastroduodenoscopy (EGD) must be fasting (at least 8 hours). Otherwise healthy patients usually require no sedation. In our unit, 90 percent of outpatients undergoing this test receive no medication other than a local anesthetic spray to the throat [lidocaine hydrochloride (Xylocaine)]. This avoids the risks attached to drug use, allows full comprehension of the findings by the patient, and permits him or her to return to work

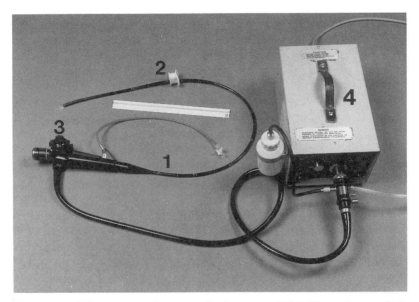

Figure 27-1. Fiberoptic esophagogastroduodenoscope (EGD). The endoscope (1) is attached to a device (4) that generates a source of illumination, suction, air pressure to inflate the stomach, and, in some cases, electrocautery. The tip of the scope is directed by control knobs (3). The delicate fiber bundle is protected by a mouthpiece (2) inserted between the teeth. The ruler is 33 centimeters (13.5 inches) in length.

soon afterward. Some anxious patients are treated with intravenous diazepam (Valium) or sublingual oxazepam. There is no justification for the risks of a general anesthetic in this procedure. In a series of more than 200,000 procedures, perforation, bleeding, infection, or cardiac events occurred in 0.13 percent. This included patients who were very ill, and the data were collected several years ago when instruments and techniques were cruder. If the procedure is done by a trained endoscopist in an otherwise healthy patient, the risk is virtually zero.

The subject is examined while lying on the left side with the chin toward the chest (Figure 27-2). After the local anesthetic spray

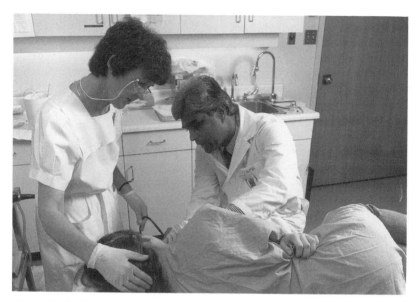

Figure 27-2. Upper gastrointestinal endoscopy (EGD). The endoscopist is introducing the gastroscope with the patient correctly positioned (note the endoscopy nurse).

is applied, the physician gently places his fingers in the throat in order to test that the spray has suppressed gagging, and to familiarize the patient with the sensation of something foreign in the anesthetized throat. One may breathe normally throughout, since the airway is not obstructed. Saliva should be allowed to drain into a provided towel. The nurse assistant urges the patient to breathe, because this helps to suppress the gag reflex. The instrument is then placed in the proper position in the throat, and the examinee is asked to swallow. Although it is difficult to swallow under these circumstances, the attempt is usually sufficient to relax the upper esophageal sphincter and allow the instrument to pass into the esophagus. A mouthpiece is placed between the teeth to protect the delicate instrument.

Once the tube is in place, the test lasts approximately 5 minutes. It is not comfortable, but there is usually no pain. The physician must inject air into the stomach in order to inflate it for better visibility, but will remove it before withdrawing the instrument. In some it may be necessary to take a biopsy of the stomach or duodenum using forceps delivered through the instrument's channel. This is painless but slightly prolongs the procedure. When the test is completed, if no sedation is given, the doctor is usually in a position to explain his findings and discuss how they might be managed.

Most IBD sufferers will not require EGD. However, Crohn's disease may affect the duodenum, and even the esophagus or stomach. If upper gut symptoms such as dyspepsia, difficulty swallowing, or heartburn occur, EGD efficiently examines these areas. Medication such as steroids or nonsteroidal antiinflammatory drugs (NSAID) may result in ulcers or esophagitis, the discovery of which requires EGD.

Fibersigmoidoscopy

The fibersigmoidoscope is shown in Figure 27-3. It is similar to the gastroscope, is about 60 centimeters in length, and is thicker to allow more suction capability. The subject should take a phosphate (Fleet) enema or similar evacuant 2 hours before the procedure. No sedation or other preparation is usually necessary. In severe diarrhea, the enema may be waived.

The procedure is performed with the patient on his left side, knees drawn up, and feet thrust forward (Figure 27-4). The doctor inspects the area around the anus for fissures, fistulas, hemorrhoids, or other perianal disease, and then gently inserts his or her index finger. The purpose is to lubricate the canal, ensure that there are no feces present, and exclude an obstructing mass. If there is a painful anal fissure (tiny tear) or other anal pathology, a local anesthetic lubricant will help.

The instrument is inserted into the rectum and maneuvered, often with the help of a nurse assistant, to its full extent, which is

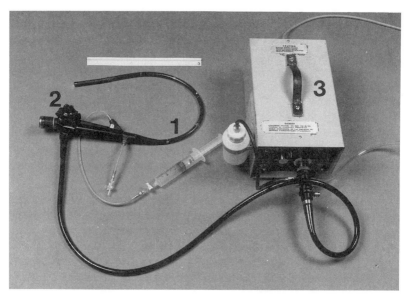

Figure 27-3. Fibersigmoidoscope (1). This instrument is shorter and thicker than the gastroscope. Note controls (2) and light source (3).

usually just short of the splenic flexure (see Figure 1-7). As a result of the presence of the instrument, the patient may be seized by an urgent need to defecate or pass gas. From Figure 1-7, the sigmoid colon can be seen to be tortuous (sigmoid means S-shaped), and the principal technical difficulty is to maneuver around it. Usually, however, the test is accomplished in about 5 minutes. Most patients do have some discomfort or pain due to looping of the instrument within the sigmoid, but comfort returns when the instrument is withdrawn. Biopsy may be done in a manner similar to that of EGD.

Sigmoidoscopy is the most important procedure in the diagnosis and management of IBD. Virtually all cases of ulcerative colitis can be identified, and biopsies taken if necessary. All the information needed to treat an acute attack and follow response to treatment can be provided by sigmoidoscopy backed up by bacteriologic examination of stool. Whether or not the disease extends beyond

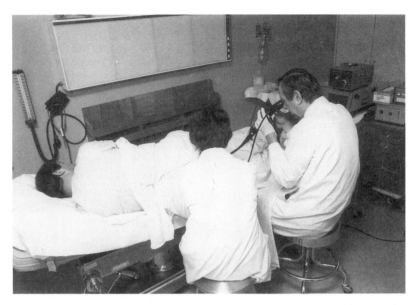

Figure 27-4. Fibersigmoidoscopy/colonoscopy. The endoscopy nurse advances the instrument while the endoscopist uses the controls. Both are able to view the colon. Some operators prefer to manage without an assistant. Newer videoscopes permit participants to observe the colon findings on a television monitor.

the reach of the instrument does not change early management. In Crohn's, the disease may lie beyond the view of the sigmoidoscope. Nevertheless, it is complementary to small-bowel x-ray and may discover Crohn's colitis.

Colonoscopy

It is possible to examine the entire colon using a *colonoscope*. This instrument resembles the fibersigmoidoscope, but is 1.6 meters in length. A full bowel preparation is necessary as for a barium enema (see the following), and sedation is frequently required. Colonoscopy takes longer than EGD or fibersigmoidoscopy and may cause more discomfort. In some cases it is not possible to maneuver the instrument right to the cecum. Colonoscopy is more costly and painful than sigmoidoscopy plus a barium enema, but permits biopsies throughout the colon. This is important in the surveillance of colons with ulcerative colitis for dysplasia or early cancer.

The patient is positioned as for fibersigmoidoscopy (Figure 27-4). Sedation is usually required. Diazepam (Valium) and meperidine hydrochloride (Demerol) are often used together. As the tip must be maneuvered around to the cecum, the procedure may be lengthy. The instrument tends to form a loop in the sigmoid colon, so that an advance at the operator's end becomes a retreat at the tip. To overcome this, the instrument is repeatedly pulled back, and abdominal pressure is exerted over the sigmoid colon. The patient may be asked to roll on his or her back, and bring up his or her knees. Sometimes the light at the tip of the colonoscope may be seen through the abdominal wall, giving a clue as to progress. The cecum is usually identified by the ileocecal valve, the opening of the appendix, and the presence of the light in the right groin. Full colonoscopy is possible in more than 80 percent of cases. In chronic ulcerative colitis, the scarred, rigid, foreshortened colon is relatively easily examined.

Colonoscopy can provide useful information in some circumstances, such as Crohn's disease confined to the right colon, or cancer surveillance. In my opinion, however, the procedure is overused. If Crohn's disease is discovered in the ileum by small-bowel x-ray, and sigmoidoscopy is normal, what difference does it make how much the cecum is involved? The exact upper margin of ulcerative colitis seldom influences management and is more cheaply and comfortably seen by barium enema. Curiosity is an insufficient indication for a costly, painful procedure in a young person already grappling with the realities of chronic illness.

Other Endoscopic Procedures

Through a side-viewing endoscope placed in the duodenum, a cannula may be passed, which is then threaded into the bile ducts or pancreatic ducts. Injected contrast material can be seen entering the duct system by x-ray. This is called *endoscopic retrograde cholangiopancreatography* (ERCP) (see Figure 16-4). It requires sedation and considerable skill on the part of the examiner. Serious complications, such as pancreatitis or cholangitis, may result. In IBD, the principal indication for ERCP is suspicion from blood tests that sclerosing cholangitis is present as an extraintestinal complication.

Enteroscopy (examination of the small bowel) may be performed with a longer endoscope, but for technical reasons it is difficult to maneuver the instrument beyond the duodenum. Even if successful, the test is too lengthy for practical use. The standard gastroscope may traverse most of the duodenum, and a good small-bowel x-ray usually detects any Crohn's in the jejunum or ileum. If the technique could be perfected, it might permit per-endoscopic stricture dilatation, thereby avoiding surgery. At operation, a surgeon may assist the endoscopist by guiding a colonoscope or enteroscope through the gut.

Rigid Sigmoidoscopy

Although reference to a tube for viewing the rectum appears in the writings of Hippocrates, the first sigmoidoscope was introduced in the late nineteenth century employing candles for illumination. It is fortunate that Edison discovered the light bulb, because colon gas may be explosive. Until recently the rigid sigmoidoscope (Figure 27-5) was the standard test for physicians wishing to examine the rectal mucosa. The instrument is relatively cheap and easy to clean and use (there are even disposable ones available). These features make it very useful in the offices of primary care physicians and surgeons where no fiberoptic equipment exists. Even in larger units, rigid sigmoidoscopy provides a quick, cheap look, permitting the physician to follow treatment effects.

The procedure may be done with no preparation or with a prior Fleet enema. It is easiest when the patient is in the knee–chest position or on a special sigmoidoscopy table. The inverted posture permits the bowel to straighten and rectal contents to fall away from the viewer. The rectum can be examined to about 15 centi-

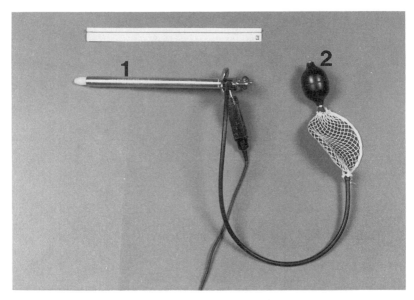

Figure 27-5. Rigid sigmoidoscope (1). Light is transmitted to the bowel by fiberoptics. The air bulb (2) allows the examiner to distend the rectum for better visibility.

meters at a sharp turn where it joins the sigmoid colon. The skilled examiner can maneuver the scope around this corner in the majority of cases, but the gain in information may not be worth the discomfort. This test is a perfectly acceptable way to follow progress in patients who have ulcerative proctitis.

BARIUM CONTRAST STUDIES

X-rays blacken photographic film. They pass through a human body, casting shadows of bones or other dense structures onto the film. The gut ordinarily casts no shadow, although air in the gut lumen can be recognized as a dark (radiolucent) area, and feces project a mottled appearance. Figure 27-6 is flat film of the abdomen showing bony structures in the transverse and sigmoid colon, and gas and feces in the cecum. In order to outline the gut, a radiopaque substance called barium is swallowed, or injected via tubes into the duodenum or rectum. X-ray pictures are then taken from various angles to detect any abnormalities of the configuration of the barium within the gut.

Upper Gastrointestinal X-ray
(Esophagus, Stomach, and Duodenum)

By swallowing barium after a fast, the patient opacifies his esophagus, stomach, and duodenum, and the shadow is projected on the x-ray film (Figure 27-7). The movement of the barium in the gut can be recorded by sequential films. Tumors appear as "filling defects" and an ulcer, as a collection of barium in the crater of the ulcer. Properly done, such x-rays detect most ulcers, tumors, and Crohn's disease, but small or diffuse lesions such as esophagitis or gastritis are difficult to see. This is not the first choice in the investigation of dyspepsia or heartburn, but will do where endoscopy is unavailable or too expensive.

Small-Bowel X-rays

It is sometimes necessary to examine the small bowel in young patients with chronic diarrhea or chronic abdominal pain, in whom Crohn's disease is suspected; that is, when there is fever, weight loss, bleeding, anemia, elevated white blood count, or a right lower abdominal mass. A *small bowel follow-through* is simply an upper gastrointestinal barium examination in which radiographs are taken as barium travels through the small bowel. Because barium becomes diluted by digestive juices as it makes its way down the gut, it is preferable to insert a tube through the nose and stomach into the

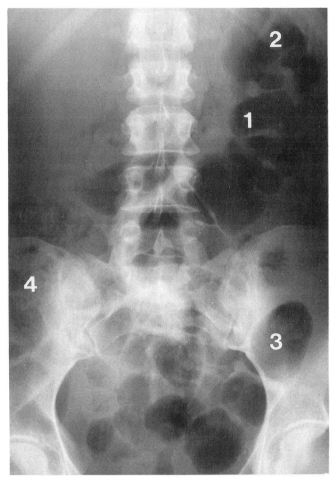

Figure 27-6. Flat film or plain x-ray of the abdomen. Air is seen in the transverse colon (1) (note haustra), splenic flexure (2), and sigmoid colon; (3) air and stool can be seen in cecum (4).

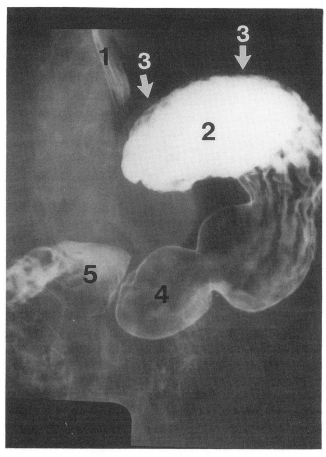

Figure 27-7. Upper gastrointestinal x-ray. Swallowed barium fills the upper gut and, on the x-ray film, outlines the esophagus (1) stomach and duodenum (5). Also shown are cardia (2) of stomach, diaphragm (3), and antrum (4) of stomach. Courtesy of Dr. H. Tao.

duodenum, through which is injected barium in a concentration that opacifies the entire small bowel. The tube is uncomfortable, but quickly removed. The test is performed more quickly than a barium swallow, and the results are far superior. This procedure is called *enteroclysis* or *small-bowel enema* (Figure 27-8). A laxative such as two bisacodyl (Dulcolax) tablets is usually taken the evening before the test.

A small-bowel enema will usually define the location and extent of small-bowel Crohn's disease. If asked, the radiologist may follow the barium into the right colon as well, perhaps obviating the need for colonoscopy or barium enema. This test also helps locate complications of Crohn's disease, such as strictures or fistulas.

Barium Enema

For this procedure, the colon must be clean, so preparation must be vigorous. Each x-ray facility has its own preference, but there are two popular techniques. The first is a fluid diet and a magnesium citrate drink at noon the day prior to the test, and enemas until the return is clear the day of the test. An increasingly popular method is the colon-washout technique accomplished by rapidly drinking 3 to 5 liters of fluid containing an osmotically effective solute such as polyethylene glycol (CoLyte, GoLYTELY) in the few hours preceding the barium enema. The doctor ordering the test should provide the patient with detailed instructions.

In the x-ray department, the radiologist inserts a small nozzle into the rectum, and barium flows into the colon by gravity. The modern air-contrast technique requires that the excess barium be evacuated once it has coated the bowel wall, and air is injected to highlight mucosal detail (Figure 27-9). The patient is asked to shift his position on the x-ray table to permit views of the various colon flexures and curves. Properly done, this is a very accurate method of detecting IBD. In early ulcerative colitis, there may be no findings, but later the featureless rigid colon, tiny ulcers, and the upper margin of disease are seen. Segments of Crohn's disease, strictures, and fistulas are best shown by this technique.

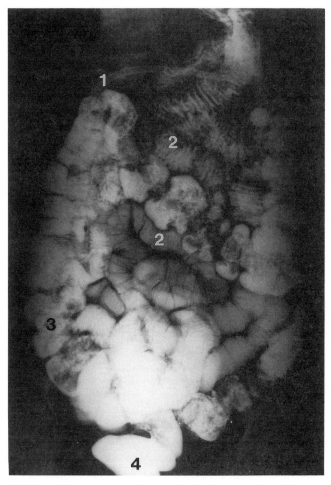

Figure 27-8. Small-bowel enema (enteroclysis). A nasogastric tube may be seen passing through stomach into the duodenum (1). Barium injected through the tube quickly opacifies the small bowel (2) to the cecum. Barium has passed into ascending colon (3) and around to rectum (4). Note the feathery appearance of the normal small bowel. Courtesy of Dr. H. Tao.

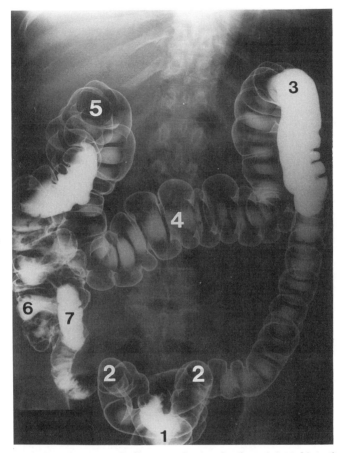

Figure 27-9. Barium enema. Radioopaque barium has been injected into the colon via a tube inserted into the rectum (1). The barium-filled colon appears white on the x-ray film. Sigmoid colon (2), splenic flexure (3), transverse colon (4) (note haustra), hepatic flexure (5), cecum (6), and terminal ileum (7) are all indicated. Courtesy of Dr. H. Tao.

ULTRASOUND OF THE ABDOMEN

Like x-rays, high-frequency sound waves penetrate the body, casting on a sensitized film or video shadows that signify structures of varying density. Unlike x-rays, sound does not damage tissue. Therefore, ultrasound is an important means by which the abdomen may be examined. Thickened loops of bowel and abscesses may be seen by this painless and harmless procedure. It is the first test to do in suspected abscess. Ultrasound is also useful to exclude gallstones in patients with episodic right upper quadrant abdominal pain, or abdominal masses that might account for lower abdominal pain. Cholesterol gallstones are prone to occur following disease, or resection of the ileum (see Chapter 14).

To undergo the test, one must be fasting. A lubricated probe is applied to and moved about the abdomen to secure images as in Figure 27-10. It is completely painless and harmless.

COMPUTERIZED TOMOGRAPHY

This remarkable technologic advance permits cross-sectional views of the body. Computerized tomography (CT) of abdomen can be very useful in Crohn's disease to detect abscesses (Figure 14-4). The thickened bowel may be identified, although strictures, small fistulas, and the extent of small-bowel involvement are best seen by small-bowel enema.

OTHER TESTS

Blood Tests

A complete blood count (CBC) includes a hemoglobin, white blood cell count, and erythrocyte sedimentation rate. The hemoglobin is the best estimation of the blood's red cell supply. If it is below normal, one is said to be anemic. Anemia may be due to bleeding, nutritional deficiency, hemolysis, or chronic inflamma-

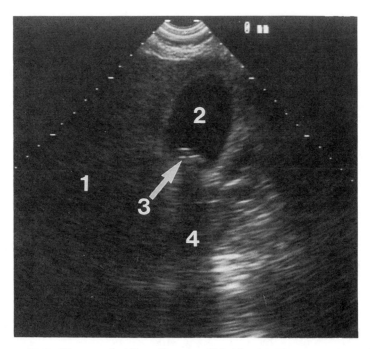

Figure 27-10. Ultrasound of liver (1) and gallbladder (2). The image shows the fluid-filled gallbladder. A gallstone (3) within the gallbladder blocks the sound waves and thus casts an *acoustic shadow* (4). This technique is 95 to 100 percent accurate in detecting gallstones in the gallbladder.

tion, all of which can occur in the angry, inflamed gut. An elevated white cell count and sedimentation rate indicate inflammation.

One may choose to do blood biochemical tests as well. Serum albumin, for example, may be low due to chronic malnutrition or protein loss from an inflamed gut. Iron, calcium, folic acid, and vitamin B_{12} levels may be included if anemia or malabsorption is suspected. When extraintestinal disease is present, tests for liver or musculoskeletal abnormalities may be necessary.

After ileal resection, vitamin B_{12} malabsorption occurs, which might, in time, cause anemia. A Schilling test assesses B_{12} absorptive capacity through a B_{12} injection to saturate liver stores, ingestion of a B_{12} pill containing a radioactive tracer, and collection of urine for 24 hours to determine how much B_{12} is absorbed and passed in the urine.

Stool Collections

Bacteriology

The organisms responsible for infectious colitis are discussed in Chapter 8. Most routine laboratories, provided with a fresh stool specimen, will identify these organisms. It is wise, however, to indicate to the lab what bacteria are likely, because this may provoke special testing. The diagnosis of antibiotic-associated or pseudomembranous colitis depends on the presence of *Clostridium difficile* toxin, not merely the presence of *C. difficile* itself.

Parasites

The parasite of principal interest in the angry gut is the ameba, *Entamoeba histolytica*. The cause of amebic dysentery, it should be searched for in travelers from the tropics with acute colitis. Other parasites may be coincidentally found in the colon, but are not recognized as pathogenetic. It is important that they not be treated as the cause of colitis. These are discussed in more detail in textbooks of parasitology or gastroenterology.

Stool Collection for Fat

If malabsorption of fat is suspected, a 3-day stool collection may be very useful. Usually, this suspicion arises when there is much small-bowel involvement with Crohn's disease, when there has been massive small-bowel resection, or when another cause of malnutrition is considered, such as bacterial overgrowth, celiac disease, or pancreatic insufficiency. The patient eats an 80-gram fat diet 24 to

48 hours prior to and during the collection. The stool is collected in a preweighed container for 72 hours commencing at 8 AM. All stools (no urine or toilet paper) must be included. The can is again weighed to determine the weight of its contents, and the stool fat is calculated. It is important that all stool produced in the 72-hour period be collected. The container should be left in a cool place and brought promptly to the lab when the collection is done.

SUMMARY

Depending on the circumstances, a minimal number of tests may be required to firmly diagnose and to estimate the severity and extent of IBD and its complications. The tests described here are relatively safe and usually only one or two are necessary. For example, sigmoidoscopy is important in ulcerative colitis, and a small-bowel enema is crucial to the diagnosis of small-bowel Crohn's disease. An upper endoscopy is helpful when one suspects upper gastrointestinal Crohn's disease or a complication of therapy, such as esophagitis or peptic ulcer. Colonoscopy or barium enema are indicated only when details of right colon involvement are important, or when cancer surveillance is required. Further tests such as CT scan, ERCP, kidney x-rays, and stool collection should be reserved for specific suspicions. Blood and stool tests for organisms are often necessary during an acute attack of IBD.

Epilogue

True hope is swift, and flies with swallow's wings;
Kings it makes gods, and meaner creatures kings.
Shakespeare, *Richard III* (ii, 15)

In these pages are found the realities of ulcerative colitis and Crohn's disease; the lifelong symptoms, the disabling complications, the difficult tests, and the unwanted effects of treatment. The recurrent and enigmatic nature of the angry gut is especially troublesome, and our ignorance of its cause offers little comfort.

Yet, despite these realities, the final message should be one of hope. For most inflammatory bowel disease (IBD) victims, there is a better day ahead. Treatment is helpful. Ulcerative colitis can be cured by surgery, and Crohn's disease can be controlled. Long-term physical disability is rare. Sex, marriage, and children are all possible. Quality of life is good, when compared to that of other chronic diseases. Many IBD patients achieve their life's aspirations; ask Rolf Benirschke and others who have made great comebacks.

There is always hope in IBD: the disease does not kill. Even when very ill, a patient should look forward to a better time. With determination and good contemporary care, nothing is impossible.

With new treatments on the horizon, an even better future seems assured. Who knows; within our lifetime, the disease itself may be conquered. Meanwhile, remember Rolf's experience:

> Maybe at first you think you never will come back, but believe me you can!

IMPORTANT ADDRESSES

Canadian Foundation for Ileitis and Colitis
National Office
21 St. Clair Avenue East, Suite 301
Toronto, Ontario M4T 1L9

Crohn's and Colitis Foundation of America
444 Park Avenue South, 11th Floor
New York, N.Y. 10018

Bibliography

CHAPTER 2

Sarna SK. Motor correlates of functional gastrointestinal symptoms. *Viewpoints Dig Dis* 1988;20:1–4.

Thompson WG. *Gut Reactions.* New York: Plenum, 1989.

CHAPTER 4

Crohn BB, Ginzburg L, Oppenheimer GD. Regional enteritis: A pathologic and clinical entity. *JAMA* 1932;99:1323–1329.

Dalziel TK. Chronic interstitial enteritis. *Br Med J* 1913;2:1068–1070.

Fielding JF. "Inflammatory" bowel disease. *Br Med J* 1985;290:47–48.

Hale-White W. Colitis. *Lancet* 1895;1:537.

Kirsner JB. Historical aspects of inflammatory bowel disease. *J Clin Gastroenterol* 1988; 10:286–297.

Myren J. Inflammatory bowel disease—a historical perspective. In: DeDombel FT, Myren J, Boucher IAD, Watkinson G, eds. *Inflammatory Bowel Disease.* London: Oxford, 1986:7–27.

Wilks S. Morbid appearances in the intestine of Miss Bankes. *Lond Med Gaz* 1859; 2:264–265.

CHAPTER 5

Binder V, Hendricksen C, Kreiner S. Prognosis in Crohn's disease—based on results from regional patient group from the county of Copenhagen. *Gut* 1985;26:146–150.

Booth IW. Chronic inflammatory bowel disease. *Arch Dis Child* 1991;66:742–744.

Hendricksen C, Kreiner S, Binder V. Long term prognosis in ulcerative colitis—based on results from a regional patient group from the county of Copenhagen. *Gut* 1985;26:158–163.

Kirsner JB, Shorter R. Recent developments in "non-specific" inflammatory bowel disease. *N Engl J Med* 1982;306:306–775.

Lindberg E, Jarnerot G, Huitfeldt B. Smoking in Crohn's disease: Effect on localization and clinical course. *Gut* 1992;33:779–782.

Meyers S, Janowitz HD. "Natural history" of Crohn's disease. An analytical review of the placebo response. *Gastroenterology* 1984;87:1189–1192.

Onions, CT (ed.). *The Shorter Oxford English Dictionary*, 3rd ed. New York: Oxford University Press, 1973.

Prior R, Gyde S, Cooke WT, Waterhouse JAH, Allan RN. Mortality in Crohn's disease. *Gastroenterology* 1981;80:307–312.

Sinclair T, Brunt PW, Mowatt NAG. Non-specific proctocolitis in northern Scotland. *Gastroenterology* 1983;85:1.

CHAPTER 6

Booth IW. Chronic inflammatory bowel disease. *Arch Dis Child* 1991;66:742–744.

Chadwick VS. Etiology of chronic ulcerative colitis and Crohn's disease. In: Phillips SF, Pemberton JH, Shorter RG, eds. *The Large Intestine*. New York: Raven Press, 1991:445–463.

Gitnick G, Challenges in inflammatory bowel diseases. In: Phillips SF, Pemberton JH, Shorter RG, eds. *The Large Intestine*. New York: Raven Press, 1991:465–475.

Kirsner JB, Shorter, R. Recent developments in "non-specific" inflammatory bowel disease. *N Engl J Med* 1982;306:306–775.

Podolsky DK. Inflammatory bowel disease (second of two parts). *N Engl J Med* 1991; 325:1008–1016.

Yamada T. *Textbook of Gastroenterology*. Philadelphia: Lippincott, 1991.

CHAPTER 7

Podolsky DK. Inflammatory bowel disease (first of two parts). *N Engl J Med* 1991; 325:928–937.

Podolsky DK. Inflammatory bowel disease (second of two parts). *N Engl J Med* 1991; 325:1008–1016.

Yamada T. *Textbook of Gastroenterology*. Philadelphia: Lippincott, 1991.

CHAPTER 8

Drossman DA, Thompson WG. Irritable bowel syndrome: A graduated, multicomponent treatment approach. *Ann Intern Med* 1992;116:1009–1016.

Guerrant RL, Bobak DA. Bacterial and protozoal gastroenteritis. *N Engl J Med* 1991; 325:327–340.

Podolsky DK. Inflammatory bowel disease (first of two parts). *N Engl J Med* 1991; 325:928–937.

Thompson WG. Gastrointestinal symptoms in the irritable bowel compared with peptic ulcer and inflammatory bowel disease. *Gut* 1984;25:1089–1092.

Yamada T. *Textbook of Gastroenterology*. Philadelphia: Lippincott, 1991.

CHAPTER 9

Courtney MG, Nunes DP, Bergin CF, et al. Randomized comparison of olsalazine and mesalamine in prevention of relapses in ulcerative colitis. *Lancet* 1992;339:1279–1281.

Dissanayake AS, Truelove SC. A controlled therapeutic trial of long-term maintenance treatment of ulcerative colitis with sulfasalazine (Salazopyrin). *Gut* 1973;14:923–926.

Jewell DP, Truelove SC. Azathioprine in ulcerative colitis: Final report on controlled clinical trial. *Br Med J* 1974;4:627–630.

Lennard-Jones JE, Longmore AJ, Newell AC, Wilson CWE, Avery-Jones F. An assessment of prednisone, Salazopyrin and topical hydrocortisone hemisuccinate used as out-patient treatment for ulcerative colitis. *Gut* 1960;1:217–222.

Lennard-Jones JE, Misciewicz JJ, Connell AM, Baron JH, Avery-Jones F. Prednisone as maintenance treatment for ulcerative colitis in remission. *Lancet* 1965;1:188–191.

Mayers S, Sachar DB, Goldberg, Janowitz HD. Corticotropin versus hydrocortisone therapy in the intravenous treatment of ulcerative colitis. *Gastroenterology* 1983; 85:351–357.

Podolsky DK. Inflammatory bowel disease (first of two parts). *N Engl J Med* 1991; 325:928–937.

Rijk MCM, Van Lier HJJ, Van Tongeren JHM. Relapse-preventing effect and safety of sulfasalazine and olsalazine in patients with ulcerative colitis in remission: A prospective, double-blind, randomized multicenter study. *Am J Med* 1992;87: 438–442.

Riley SA, Mani V, Goodman MJ, et al. Comparison of delayed release 5-aminosalicylic acid (Mesalazine) and sulfasalazine as maintenance treatment for patients with ulcerative colitis. *Gastroenterology* 1988;94:1383–1389.

Truelove SC, Witts LJ. Cortisone in ulcerative colitis. *Br Med J* 1955;3:1041–1048.

Truelove, SC, Witts LJ. Cortisone and corticotropin in ulcerative colitis. *Br Med J* 1959; 1:387–394.

CHAPTER 10

Booth IW. Chronic inflammatory bowel disease. *Arch Dis Child* 1991;66:742–744.
Podolsky DK. Inflammatory bowel disease (second of two parts). *N Engl J Med* 1991;325:1008–1016.
Yamada T. *Textbook of Gastroenterology*. Philadelphia: Lippincott, 1991.

CHAPTER 11

Crohn BB, Ginzburg L, Oppenheimer GD. Regional enteritis: A pathologic and clinical entity. *JAMA* 1932;99:1323–1329.
Dalziel TK. Chronic interstitial enteritis. *Br Med J* 1913;2:1068–1070.
Yamada T. *Textbook of Gastroenterology*. Philadelphia: Lippincott, 1991.

CHAPTER 12

Admans H, Whorwell PJ, Wright R. Diagnosis of Crohn's disease. *Dig Dis Sci* 1980; 25:911–915.
Booth IW. Chronic inflammatory bowel disease. *Arch Dis Child* 1991;66:742–744.
Gitnick G. Challenges in inflammatory bowel diseases. In: Phillips SF, Pemberton JH, Shorter RG, eds. *The Large Intestine*. New York: Raven Press, 1991;465–475.
Puntis J, McNeish AS, Allan RN. Long term prognosis of Crohn's disease with onset in childhood and adolescence. *Gut* 1984;25:329–336.
Thompson WG. Gastrointestinal symptoms in the irritable bowel compared with peptic ulcer and inflammatory bowel disease. *Gut* 1984;25:1089–1092.
Yamada T. *Textbook of Gastroenterology*. Philadelphia: Lippincott, 1991.

CHAPTER 13

Ewe K, Kerbach U. Factitious diarrhea. *Clin Gastroenterol* 1986;15:723–740.
Lashner BA. Incorporating randomized clinical trials into clinical practice: Maintenance treatment for Crohn's disease. *Am J Gastroenterol* 1992;87:549–550.
Malchow H, Ewe K, Brandes JW, *et al.* European cooperative Crohn's disease study (ECCDS): Results of drug treatment. *Gastroenterology* 1984;86:249–266.
O'Morain C, Segal AW, Levi AJ. Elemental diet as primary treatment of acute Crohn's disease. *Br Med J* 1984;288:1859–1862.
Prantera C, Pallone F, Brunetti G, Cottone M, Miglioli M. Oral 5-aminosalicylic acid (Asacol) in the maintenance treatment of Crohn's disease. *Gastroenterology* 1992;103:363–368.

Present DH, Korelitz BI, Wisch N, Glass JL, Sachar DB, Pasternack BS. Treatment of Crohn's disease with 6-mercaptopurine; a long-term, randomized double-blind study. *N Engl J Med* 1980;302:981–987.

Rijk MCM, Van Hogezand RA, Van Lier HJJ, Van Tongeren JHM. Sulfasalazine and prednisone compared with prednisone for treating active Crohn's disease. *Ann Intern Med* 1991;114:445–450.

Salomon P, Kornbluth A, Aisenberg J, Janowitz HD. How effective are current drugs for Crohn's disease? A meta-analysis. *J Clin Gastroenterol* 1992;14:211–215.

Singleton JW, Law DH, Kelley ML, Mekhjian HS, Sturdevant RAL. National Cooperative Crohn's Disease Study: Adverse reactions to study drugs. *Gastroenterology* 1979;77:870–882.

Singleton JW, Summers RW, Kern F, *et al.* A trial of sulfasalazine as adjunctive therapy in Crohn's disease. *Gastroenterology* 1979;77:887–897.

Summers RW, Switz DM, Sessions JT, *et al.* National Cooperative Crohn's Disease Study: Results of drug treatment. *Gastroenterology* 1979;77:847–869.

Tremaine WJ. Maintenance of remission in Crohn's disease: is 5'-aminosalicylic acid the answer? *Gastroenterology* 1992;103:694–704.

Ursing B, Alm T, Barang F, *et al.* A comparative study of metronidazole and sulfasalazine for active Crohn's disease: The cooperative Crohn's disease study in Sweden. II Result. *Gastroenterology* 1982; 83:550–562.

CHAPTER 14

Booth IW. Chronic inflammatory bowel disease. *Arch Dis Child* 1991;66:742–744.

Podolsky DK. Inflammatory bowel disease (second of two parts). *N Engl J Med* 1991;325:1008–1016.

Puntis J, McNeish AS, Allan RN. Long term prognosis of Crohn's disease with onset in childhood and adolescence. *Gut* 1984;25:329–336.

Yamada T. *Textbook of Gastroenterology.* Philadelphia: Lippincott, 1991.

CHAPTER 15

de Silva HJ, Millard PR, Soper N, Kettlewell M, Mortensen N, Jewell DP. Effects of the fecal stream and stasis on the ileal pouch mucosa. *Gut* 1991;32:1166–1169.

Harig JM, Soergel KH, Komorowski RA, Wood CM. Treatment of diversion colitis with short-chain fatty acid irrigation. *N Engl J Med* 1989;320:23–28.

Jessurun J, Yardley JH, Giardiello FM, Hamilton SL, Bayless TM. Chronic colitis with thickening of the subepithelial collagen layer (collagenous colitis). *Hum Pathol* 1987;18:839–848.

Kingham JG. Microscopic colitis. *Gut* 1991;32:234–235.

Lazenby AJ, Yardley JH, Giardiello FM, Jessurun J, Bayless TM. Lymphocytic (microscopic colitis). *Hum Pathol* 1989;20:18–28.

Lazenby AJ, Yardley JH, Giardiello FM, Jessurun J, Bayless TM. Lymphocytic ("microscopic") colitis: A comparative histopathologic study with particular reference to collagenous colitis. *Hum Pathol* 1987;20:18–28.

Lee E, Schiller L, Vandrell D, Santa Ana CA, Fortran JS. Subepithelial collagen table thickness in colon specimens from patients with microscopic colitis and collagenous colitis. *Gastroenterology* 1992;103:1790–1796.

McIntosh D, Thompson WG, Patel D, Barr JR, Guindi M. Is rectal biopsy necessary in irritable bowel syndrome? *Am J Gastroenterol* 1992;87:1407–1409.

Peppercorn MA. Drug-responsive chronic segmental colitis associated with diverticula: A clinical syndrome in the elderly. *Am J Gastroenterol* 1992;87:609–612.

Pockros PJ, Foroozan P. GoLYTELY lavage versus a standard colonoscopy preparation: Effect on normal colonic mucosal histology. *Gastroenterology* 1985;88:545–548.

Podolsky DK. Inflammatory bowel disease (first of two parts). *N Engl J Med* 1991;325:928–937.

Rauh SM, Schoetz DJ, Roberts PL, Murray JJ, Collat JA, Veidenheimer MC. Pouchitis—is it a wastebasket diagnosis? *Dis Colon Rectum* 1991;34:685–689.

Smith GE, Kime LR, Pitcher JL. The colitis of Behçet's disease: A separate entity. *Dig Dis Sci* 1973;18:987–1000.

Tanaka M, Mazzolini G, Riddell RH. Distribution of collagenous colitis. *Gut* 1992;33:65–70.

Thompson WG. *The Irritable Gut*. Baltimore: University Park Press, 1979, Chap. 19, pp. 281–305.

CHAPTER 16

Allan RN. Extraintestinal manifestations of inflammatory bowel disease. *Clin Gastroenterol* 1988;12:617–632.

Danzi JT. Extraintestinal manifestations of idiopathic inflammatory bowel disease. *Arch Intern Med* 1992;148:297–302.

Farrant JM, Hayllar KM, Wilkinson ML, *et al.* Natural history and prognostic variables in primary sclerosing cholangitis. *Gastroenterology* 1991;100:1710–1717.

Gravellese EM, Kantrowitz FG. Arthritic manifestations of inflammatory bowel disease. *Am J Gastroenterol* 1988;83:703–709.

Kraft SC. Crohn's disease of the mouth. *Ann Intern Med* 1975;83:570–571.

Mir-Madjlessi SH, Taylor JS, Farmer RG. Clinical course and evolution of erythema nodosum and pyoderma gangrenosum in chronic ulcerative colitis: A study of 42 patients. *Am J Gastroenterol* 1985;80:615–620.

Olsson R, Danielsson A, Jarnerot G, *et al.* Prevalence of primary sclerosing cholangitis in patients with ulcerative colitis. *Gastroenterology* 1991;100: 1319–1323.

Podolsky DK. Inflammatory bowel disease (second of two parts). *N Engl J Med* 1991; 325:1008–1016.

Rankin GB. Extraintestinal and systemic manifestations of inflammatory bowel disease. *Med Clin North Am* 1990;74:39–50.

Whorwell PJ, Hawkins R, Dewbury K, *et al.*. Ultrasound survey of gallstones and other hepatobiliary disorders in patients with Crohn's disease. *Dig Dis Sci* 1984; 29:930.

Yamada T. *Textbook of Gastroenterology.* Philadelphia: Lippincott, 1991.

CHAPTER 17

Baker WNW, Glass RE, Ritchie JK, Aylett SO. Cancer of the rectum following colectomy and ileorectal anastomosis for ulcerative colitis. *Br J Surg* 1978;65:862–868.

DeDombel FT, Watts JM, Watkinson G, Goligher JC. Local complications of ulcerative colitis: Stricture, pseudopolyposis, and carcinoma of the colon and rectum. *Br Med J* 1966;1:1442–1447.

Devroede CH, Tayler WF. On calculating cancer risk and survival of ulcerative colitis patients with the life table method. *Gastroenterology* 1976;71:505–509.

Greenstein AJ, Sachar DB, Smith H, *et al.* Cancer in universal and left-sided ulcerative colitis: Factors determining risk. *Gastroenterology* 1979;77:290–294.

Grundfest SF, Fazio V, Weiss RA, *et al.* The risk of cancer following colectomy and ileorectal anastomosis for extensive ulcerative colitis. *Ann Surg* 1981;193:9–14.

Hendricksen C, Kreiner S, Binder V. Long term prognosis in ulcerative colitis—based on results from a regional patient group from the county of Copenhagen. *Gut* 1985;26:158–163.

Maratka Z, Nedbal J, Kocianova J, Havelka J, Kudrmann J, Hendl J. Incidence of colorectal cancer in proctocolitis: A retrospective study of 959 cases over 40 years. *Gut* 1985;26:43–49.

Senay E, Sachar DB, Keohane M, Greenstein AJ. Small bowel carcinoma in Crohn's disease: Distinguishing features and risk factors. *Cancer* 1989;63:360–363.

Stenson WF, MacDermott RP. Inflammatory bowel disease. In: Yamada T, ed. *Textbook of Gastroenterology.* Philadelphia: Lippincott, 1991:1588–1645.

Thompson WG, Gillies RR, Silver HKB, Schuster J, Freedman SO, Gold P. Carcinoembryonic antigen and alpha 1-fetoprotein in ulcerative colitis and regional enteritis. *Can Med Assoc J* 1974;110:775–777.

CHAPTER 18

Drossman DA, Leserman J, Li Z, Mitchell CM, Zagami EA, Patrick DL. The rating form of IBD patient concerns: A new measure of health status. *Psychosom Med* 1991;53:701–712.

Drossman DA, Leserman J, Mitchell CM, Li Z, Zagami EA, Patrick DL. Health status and health care use in persons with inflammatory bowel disease: A national sample. *Dig Dis Sci* 1991;36:1746–1755.

Drossman DA, Patrick DL, Mitchell CM, Zagami EW, Appelbaum MI. health related quality of life in inflammatory bowel disease: Functional status and patient worries and concerns. *Dig Dis Sci* 1989;34:1379–1386.

Farmer RG, Easley KA, Farmer JM. Quality of life assessment by patients with inflammatory bowel disease. *Cleve Clin J Med* 1992;59:35–42.

Hendriksen C, Binder V. Social prognosis in patients with ulcerative colitis. *Br Med J* 1980;2:581–583.

Levenstein S, Prantera C, Varvo V, *et al*. Stress, symptoms and rectal inflammation in ulcerative colitis. *Gastroenterology* 1992;102:A474.

Mayberry MK, Probert C, Srivastava E, Rhodes J, Mayberry JF. Perceived discrimination in education and employment by people with Crohn's disease: A case control study of educational achievement and employment. *Gut* 1992;33:312–314.

North CS, Alpers DH, Helzer JE, Spitznagel EL, Clouse RE. Do life events or depression exacerbate inflammatory bowel disease? *Ann Intern Med* 1991;114;381–386.

Sorensen VZ, Olsen BG, Binder V. Life prospects and quality of life in patients with Crohn's disease. *Gut* 1987;28:382–385.

Vallis TM, Turnbull GK. Clinical management of inflammatory bowel disease; Beyond disease activity. 1. Assessing psychosocial factors 2. *Can J Gastroenterol* 1992;6:39–43.

CHAPTER 19

Baiocco PC, Korelitz BI. The influence of inflammatory bowel disease and its treatment on pregnancy and fetal outcome. *J Clin Gastroenterol* 1984;6:211–216.

Jarnerpt G, Into-Malmberg MB. Sulfasalazine treatment during breast feeding. *Scand J Gastroenterol* 1979;14:869–871.

Levi AJ, Fisher AM, Hughes L. Hendry WF. Male infertility due to sulfasalazine. *Lancet* 1979;2:276–278.

Mogadam M, Dobbins WO III, Korelitz BI. The safety of corticosteroids, and sulfasalazine in pregnancy associated with inflammatory bowel disease. *Gastroenterology* 1980;78:1224.

Singer AJ, Brandt LJ. Pathophysiology of the gastrointestinal tract during pregnancy. *Am J Gastroenterol* 1991;86:1695–1712.

Willoughby CP, Truelove SC. Ulcerative colitis and pregnancy. *Gut* 1980;21:469–474.

CHAPTER 20

Courtney MG, Nunes DP, Bergin CF, *et al.*. Randomized comparison of olsalazine and mesalamine in prevention of relapses in ulcerative colitis. *Lancet* 1992;339:1279–1281.

Dissanayake AS, Truelove SC. A controlled therapeutic trial of long-term maintenance treatment of ulcerative colitis with sulfasalazine (Salazopyrin). *Gut* 1973;14: 923–926.

Lashner BA. Incorporating randomized clinical trials into clinical practice: Maintenance treatment for Crohn's disease. *Am J Gastroenterol* 1992;87:549–550.

Lennard-Jones JE, Longmore AJ, Newell AC, Wilson CWE, Avery-Jones F. An assessment of prednisone, Salazopyrin and topical hydrocortisone hemisuccinate used as out-patient treatment for ulcerative colitis. *Gut* 1960;1:217–222.

Misciewicz JJ, Lennard-Jones JE, Connell AM, Baron JH, Avery-Jones F. Controlled trial of sulfasalazine in maintenance therapy for ulcerative colitis. *Lancet* 1965; 1:185–188.

Prantera C, Pallone F, Brunetti G, Cottone M, Miglioli M. Oral 5-aminosalicylic acid (Asacol) in the maintenance treatment of Crohn's disease. *Gastroenterology* 1992; 103:363–368.

Rijk MCM, Van Hogezand RA, Van Lier HJJ, Van Tongeren JHM. Sulfasalazine and prednisone compared with prednisone for treating active Crohn's disease. *Ann Intern Med* 1991;114:445–450.

Rijk MCM, Van Lier HJJ, Van Tongeren JHM. Relapse-preventing effect and safety of sulfasalazine and olsalazine in patients with ulcerative colitis in remission: A prospective, double-blind, randomized multicenter study. *Am J Med* 1992;87: 438–442.

Singleton JW, Law DH, Kelley ML, Mekhjian HS, Sturdevant RAL. National Cooperative Crohn's Disease Study: Adverse reactions to study drugs. *Gastroenterology* 1979;77:870–882.

Singleton JW, Summers RW, Kern F, et al. A trial of sulfasalazine as adjunctive therapy in Crohn's disease. *Gastroenterology* 1979;77:887–897.

Summers RW, Switz DM, Sessions JT, et al. National Cooperative Crohn's Disease Study: Results of drug treatment. *Gastroenterology* 1979;77:847–869.

Svartz N. The treatment of 124 cases of ulcerative colitis with Salazopyrin and attempts at desensitization in cases of hypersensitization to sulfa. *Acta Med Scand* 1948;206(suppl):465–472.

Tremaine WJ. Maintenance of remission in Crohn's disease: Is 5'-aminosalicylic acid the answer? *Gastroenterology* 1992;103:694–696.

CHAPTER 21

Lennard-Jones JE, Longmore AJ, Newell AC, Wilson CWE, Avery-Jones F. An assessment of prednisone, Salazopyrin and topical hydrocortisone hemisuccinate used as out-patient treatment for ulcerative colitis. *Gut* 1960;1:217–222.

Lennard-Jones JE, Misciewicz JJ, Connell AM, Baron JH, Avery-Jones F. Prednisone as maintenance treatment for ulcerative colitis in remission. *Lancet* 1965;1:188–191.

Melchow H, Ewe K, Brandes JW, et al. European Cooperative Crohn's Disease Study (ECCDS). *Gastroenterology* 1984;86:249–266.

Summers RW, Switz DM, Sessions JT, et al. National Cooperative Crohn's Disease Study: Results of drug treatment. *Gastroenterology* 1979;77:847–869.

Truelove SC, Witts LJ. Cortisone in ulcerative colitis. *Br Med J* 1955;3:1041–1048.

Truelove SC, Witts LJ. Cortisone and corticotropin in ulcerative colitis. *Br Med J* 1959; 1:387–394.

CHAPTER 22

Dollery S (ed). *Therapeutic Drugs*. London: Churchill Livingstone, 1991.

Archambeault A, Feagan B, Fedorak R, et al. The Canadian Crohn's relapse prevention trial. *Gastroenterology* 1992;102:A591.

Brynskov J, Freund L, Rasmussen SN, et al. A placebo-controlled, double-blind, randomized trial of cyclosporine therapy in active chronic Crohn's disease. *N Engl J Med* 1989;321;845–850.

Gitnick G. Challenges in inflammatory bowel diseases. In: Phillips SF, Pemberton JH, Shorter RG, eds. *The Large Intestine*. New York: Raven Press, 1991:465–475.

Janowitz HD, Bilotta JJ. Critical evaluation of the medical therapy of inflammatory bowel disease. In: Phillips SF, Pemberton JH, Shorter RG, eds. *The Large Intestine*. New York: Raven Press, 1991;475–500.

Jewell DP, Truelove SC. Azathioprine in ulcerative colitis; final report on controlled clinical trial. *Br Med J* 1974;4:627–630.

Kozarek RA, Patterson DJ, Gelfand MD, Botoman VA, Ball T, Wilske KR. Methotrexate induces clinical and histologic remission in patients with refractory inflammatory bowel disease. *Ann Intern Med* 1989;10:353–356.

Melchow H, Ewe K, Brandes JW, et al. European Cooperative Crohn's Disease Study (ECCDS). *Gastroenterology* 1984;86:249–266.

Podolsky DK. Inflammatory bowel disease (second of two parts). *N Engl J Med* 1991;325:1008–1016.

Present DH, Korelitz BI, Wisch N, Glass JL, Sachar DB, Pasternack BS. Treatment of Crohn's disease with 6-mercaptopurine: A long-term, randomized double-blind study. *N Engl J Med* 1980;302:981–987.

Stenson WF, MacDermott RP. Inflammatory bowel disease. In: Yamada T, ed. *Textbook of Gastroenterology*. Philadelphia: Lippincott, 1991:1588–1645.

Summers RW, Switz DM, Sessions JT, et al. National Cooperative Crohn's Disease Study: Results of drug treatment. *Gastroenterology* 1979;77:847–869.

CHAPTER 23

Dollery S (ed). *Therapeutic Drugs*. London: Churchill Livingstone, 1991.

Bernstein LH, Frank MS, Brandt LJ, Boley SJ. Healing perianal Crohn's disease with metronidazole. *Gastroenterology* 1980;79:357–365.

Janowitz DH, Bilotta JJ, Critical evaluation of the medical therapy of inflammatory bowel disease. In: Phillips SF, Pemberton JH, Shorter RG, eds. *The Large Intestine.* New York: Raven Press, 1991:475–500.

Podolsky DK. Inflammatory bowel disease (first of two parts). *N Engl J Med* 1991; 325:928–937.

Sutherland L, Singleton J, Sessions J, et al. Double blind, placebo controlled trial of metronidazole in Crohn's disease. *Gut* 1991;32:1071–1075.

Ursing B, Alm T, Barany F, et al. A comparative study of metronidazole and sulfasalazine for active Crohn's disease: The cooperative Crohn's disease study in Sweden. II. Result. *Gastroenterology* 1992;83:550–562.

CHAPTER 24

Archambeault A, Feagan B, Fedorak R, et al. The Canadian Crohn's relapse prevention trial. *Gastroenterology* 1992;102:A591.

Baron JH, Connell AM, Lennard-Jones JE, Avery-Jones F. Sulfasalazine and salicylazosulfadimidine in ulcerative colitis. *Lancet* 1962;1:1094–1096.

Best WR, Becktel JM, Singleton JW, Kern F Jr. Development of a Crohn's disease activity index. National Cooperative Crohn's Disease Study. *Gastroenterology* 1976; 70:439–444.

Brody H. The lie that heals: The ethics of giving placebos. *Ann Intern Med* 1982;97: 112–118.

Brynskov J, Freund L, Rasmussen SN, et al. A placebo-controlled, double-blind, randomized trial of cyclosporine therapy in active chronic Crohn's disease. *N Engl J Med* 1989;381:845–850.

Courtney MG, Nunes DP, Bergin CF, et al. Randomized comparison of olsalazine and mesalamine in prevention of relapses in ulcerative colitis. *Lancet* 1992;339:1279–1281.

Dissanayake AS, Truelove SC. A controlled therapeutic trial of long-term maintenance treatment of ulcerative colitis with sulfasalazine (Salazopyrin). *Gut* 1973;14: 923–926.

Dollery S (ed). *Therapeutic Drugs.* London: Churchill Livingstone, 1991.

Jewell DP, Truelove SC. Azathioprine in ulcerative colitis; final report on controlled clinical trial. *Br Med J* 1974;4:627–630.

Lennard-Jones JE, Longmore AJ, Newell AC, Wilson CWE, Avery-Jones F. An assessment of prednisone, Salazopyrin and topical hydrocortisone hemisuccinate used as out-patient treatment for ulcerative colitis. *Gut* 1960;1:217–222.

Lind J. *A Treatise of the Scurvy.* Edinburgh: University Press, 1953.

Melchow H, Ewe K, Brandes JW, et al. European Cooperative Crohn's Disease Study (ECCDS). *Gastroenterology* 1984;86:249–266.

Meyers S, Janowitz HD. "Natural history" of Crohn's disease. An analytical review of the placebo response. *Gastroenterology* 1984;87:1189–1192.

Misciewicz JJ, Lennard-Jones JE, Connell AM, Baron JH, Avery-Jones F. Controlled trial of sulfasalazine in maintenance therapy for ulcerative colitis. *Lancet* 1965; 1:185–188.

O'Donoghue DP, Dawson AM, Powell-Tuck J, Bown RL, Lennard-Jones JE. Double-blind withdrawal trial of azathioprine as maintenance treatment for Crohn's disease. *Lancet* 1978;2:955–957.

Prantera C, Pallone F, Brunetti G, Cottone M, Miglioli M. Oral 5-aminosalicylic acid (Asacol) in the maintenance treatment of Crohn's disease. *Gastroenterology* 1992; 103:363–368.

Present DH, Korelitz BI, Wisch N, Glass JL, Sachar DB, Pasternack BS. Treatment of Crohn's disease with 6-mercaptopurine; a long-term, randomized double-blind study. *N Engl J Med* 1980;302:981–987.

Rijk MCM, Van Hogezand RA, Van Lier HJJ, Van Tongeren JHM. Sulfasalazine and prednisone compared with prednisone for treating active Crohn's disease. *Ann Intern Med* 1991;114:445–450.

Rijk MCM, Van Lier HJJ, Van Tongeren JHM. Relapse-preventing effect and safety of sulfasalazine and olsalazine in patients with ulcerative colitis in remission: A prospective, double-blind, randomized multicenter study. *Am J Med* 1992;87: 438–442.

Riley SA, Mani V, Goodman MJ, *et al.* Comparison of delayed release 5-aminosalicylic acid (Mesalazine) and sulfasalazine as maintenance treatment for patients with ulcerative colitis. *Gastroenterology* 1988;94:1383–1389.

Singleton JW, Summers RW, Kern F, *et al.* A trial of sulfasalazine as adjunctive therapy in Crohn's disease. *Gastroenterology* 1979;77:887–897.

Summers RW, Switz DM, Sessions JT, *et al.* National cooperative Crohn's disease study: Results of drug treatment. *Gastroenterology* 1979;77:847–869.

Svartz N. The treatment of 124 cases of ulcerative colitis with Salazopyrin and attempts at desensitization in cases of hypersensitization to sulfa. *Acta Med Scand* 1948;206(suppl):465–472.

Tremaine WJ. Maintenance of remission in Crohn's disease: Is 5'-aminosalicylic acid the answer? *Gastroenterology* 1992;103:694–696.

Truelove SC, Witts LJ. Cortisone in ulcerative colitis. *Br Med J* 1955;3:1041–1048.

Truelove SC, Witts LJ. Cortisone and corticotropin in ulcerative colitis. *Br Med J* 1959; 1:387–394.

Ursing B, Alm T, Barang F, *et al.* A comparative study of metronidazole and sulfasalazine for active Crohn's disease: The cooperative Crohn's disease study in Sweden. II Result. *Gastroenterology* 1982;83:550–562.

CHAPTER 25

Dickenson RJ, Ashton MG, Axon AT, Hill GL. Controlled trial of intravenous hyperalimentation and total bowel rest as an adjunct to the routine therapy of acute colitis. *Gastroenterology* 1980;79:1199–1204.

Greenberg GR, Fleming CR, Jeejeebhoy KN, Rosenberg IH, Sales D, Tremaine WJ. Controlled trial of bowel rest and nutritional support in the management of Crohn's disease. *Gut* 1988;29:1309–1315.

Lochs H, Steinhardt HJ, Klaus-Wentz B, Zeitz M. Comparison of enteral nutrition and drug treatment in active Crohn's disease. Study IV. *Gastroenterology* 1991;101:881–888.

Morin CL, Roulet M, Roy CC, Weber A. Continuous elemental enteral alimentation in children with Crohn's disease and growth failure. *Gastroenterology* 1980;79:1205–1210.

O'Morain C, Segal AW, Levi AJ. Elemental diet as primary treatment of acute Crohn's disease. *Br Med J* 1984;288:1859–1862.

CHAPTER 26

Greenstein AJ, Sachar DB, Pasternack BS, Janowitz HD. Reoperation and recurrence in Crohn's colitis and ileocolitis: crude and cumulative rates. *N Engl J Med* 1975; 293:685–690.

Lock MR, Farmer RG, Fazio VW, Jagelman DG, Lavery IC, Weakley FL. Recurrence and reoperation for Crohn's disease: The role of disease location in prognosis. *N Engl J Med* 1981;304:1586–1588.

Olaison G, Smedh K, Sjodahl R. Natural course of Crohn's disease after ileocolic resection: Endoscopically visualized ileal ulcers preceding symptoms. *Gut* 1992; 33:331–335.

Pallone F, Boirivant M, Stazi MA, Cosintino R, Prantera C, Torsoli A. Analysis of clinical course of postoperative Crohn's disease of distal ileum. *Dig Dis Sci* 1992; 37:215–219.

Parks A, Beliveau P. Proctocolectomy with ileal reservoir and anal anastomosis. *Br J Surg* 1980;67:533–538.

Pemberton JH. Surgical approaches to proctocolectomy for inflammatory bowel disease. In: Phillips SF, Shorter RG, Pemberton JH, eds. *The Large Intestine: Physiology, Pathophysiology and Disease.* New York: Raven Press; 1991:629–655.

Thompson WG, Wrathell E. The relation between ileal resection and vitamin B_{12} absorption. *Can J Surg* 1977;20:461–464.

Tse GN, Beattie WG, Thompson WG. Incidence of diarrhea following ileal resection. *Can J Surg* 1972;15:3–4.

Index